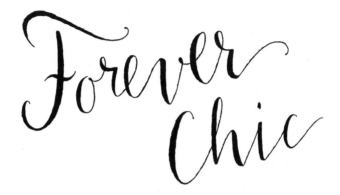

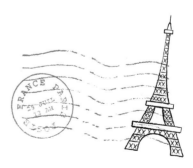

First published in the United States of America in 2013

by Rizzoli Ex Libris, an imprint of

Rizzoli International Publications, Inc.

300 Park Avenue South

New York, NY 10010

www.rizzoliusa.com

MEDICAL DISCLAIMER: This book is not intended as a substitute
for the medical advice of physicians. As always, please consult with
your doctor before beginning any diet or supplement regimen.

2013 2014 2015 2016 / 10 9 8 7 6 5 4 3 2 1

Distributed in the U.S. trade by Random House, New York

Printed in China

ISBN-13: 978-0-8478-4149-3

Library of Congress Catalog Control Number: 2013939260

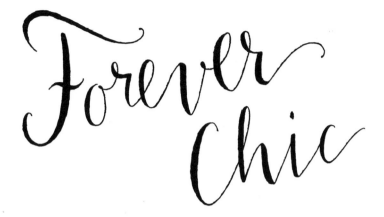

Forever Chic

Frenchwomen's Secrets for Timeless Beauty, Style *and* Substance

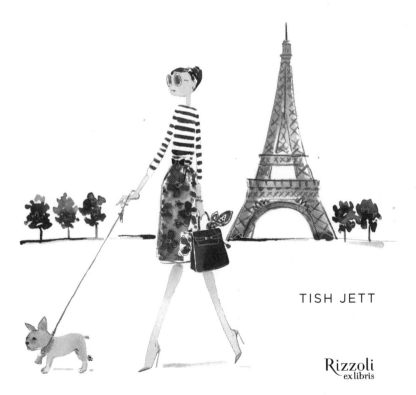

TISH JETT

Rizzoli
ex libris

FOR ALEXANDRE AND ANDREA.
Always.

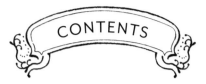

CONTENTS

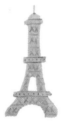

PREFACE

What's Age Got to Do with It?

"This is the program," I told my eight-year-old daughter, Andrea. "We're moving to France for two years!" I was going for my dream job as style editor of the *International Herald Tribune*.

"I'm not coming," Andrea said.

"Oh, but it will be wonderful!" I explained, my voice almost giddy. "You'll learn to speak French and have one of the most extraordinary experiences of your life! You can get a French cat! You'll thank me one day."

Since we didn't live in a domestic democracy, Andrea said goodbye to her friends in Bedford, New York, and I arranged for our three very large dogs, adopted from our local humane society, to be on our flight, and we set off on our excellent French adventure.

Occasionally, best-laid plans turn out to be better than one expects, as in moving for a job and staying for love. Talk about a win-win. I met the love of my life at one of those splendid French dinner parties. The thoughtful hostess had invited an exceedingly attractive single Frenchman who spoke fluent English. That fluent English was key, because when I met the man who is now my husband and my reason for living in France, my French vocabulary consisted at best of twenty words, mostly unconnected by verbs.

That was more than twenty-five years ago.

To my astonishment, in those decades, I went from thirtysomething to something entirely unexpected: a *femme d'un certain âge*.

And never had I anticipated a bonus on the horizon: women of a certain age and even of "*un âge certain*" (as my first and best French friend, Anne-Françoise de Saint Seine-Henner, says) are considered alluring, mysterious, and seductive in France.

That's why, from my up-close and personal point of view, I'm living in a woman's wonderland.

Early on, I realized I had an unprecedented opportunity: I could use my exposure to the masters to learn about timeless elegance.

I set out to discover how my role models aged with grace and singular style while seemingly never obsessing about the passage of time, concentrating solely on looking their best while taking care of themselves, which also means eating well, watching their weight, drinking little, exercising, and fiercely celebrating lives well lived.

After a brief internal debate about reconciling façade and substance, I realized they are inseparable. That's what the French call *bien-être,* or well-being, which in its full translation means creating harmony in one's life. I came to the conclusion that spending fifteen to twenty minutes preparing for each new day is worth every second.

The first part of my learning experience came with understanding the precept that looking good is the best revenge. Age has nothing to do with it. Self-respect and pleasure have everything to do with it.

When the façade is firmly in place, a woman becomes confident, and what's more attractive than confidence? Frenchwomen of all ages are admired for their legendary poise and presence. These qualities alone transform the simplest clothes into a look of natural chic. Never do they appear stilted, contrived, or consciously put together. Nor do they give the impression that a great deal of effort went into pulling together their looks, even—perhaps especially—on occasions when it did.

The second part of their secret, which makes them even more inspiring, is that while constantly polishing, pampering, and perfecting their exteriors, they're hard at work enhancing and maintaining their internal resources. Façade, though a function of their personalities, is never enough.

Wit, charm, and informed intelligence are the coins of the realm. Add elegance to the mix, and the result is an intoxicating cocktail of fascinating femininity.

Imagine a woman who has read the latest books, seen the newest international films, and visited the current exhibitions and knows how to toss a soupçon of historical trivia into a conversation. Irresistible, *non*?

Remaining sublimely intriguing throughout one's life may be an art, but it is one any woman can learn. I'm a work in progress. And in these pages, I will tell you everything I know.

So what if the last time we saw forty it was on a speedometer? *Ç'est la vie.*

It's not about the numbers. No one knows this better than Frenchwomen. Living a beautiful life is about style, simplicity, intelligence, and generosity. It's about a singularly unique blend of realism and *joie de vivre*. Life has its unavoidable complications (again, realism), but that never precludes an appreciation and celebration of the joys of life.

Forever Chic is dedicated to women forty-ish to whatever-ish, and every detail herein has been chosen for you—for us—to wear, to use, to amuse. Even better, someone, namely *moi*, has tried and tested every trick, secret, product, discipline, snippet of advice, and wardrobe wonder that is explained in detail in these pages.

Stay with me and I guarantee you will rethink age, beauty, well-being, and style. Together we are about to embark on a life-enhancing cultural-exchange program with the masters of looking extraordinary forever, *les femmes françaises d'un certain âge.*

Welcome to my world and *merci par avance* for joining me.

The Allure of *La Femme Française d'Un Certain Âge*

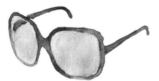

When I'm asked, as I inevitably am, to explain the elusive style and beauty secrets that Frenchwomen of a certain age all seem to possess, I respond with a resounding "*Absolument!*"

After more than two decades of total immersion in the culture, I have figured out and stolen (excuse me, appropriated) many of the remarkable practices that allow Frenchwomen to seemingly transcend age and appear youthful, vibrant, and stylish throughout their lives.

It's taken time and intensive study, bordering on obsession, I admit, but I finally understand the famous phrase *je ne sais quoi* that everyone employs to explain what Frenchwomen have and we (reputedly) don't. Let me assure you that we, too, can have that inexplicable something. Read on.

WHAT IS SO SPECIAL ABOUT FRENCHWOMEN OF A CERTAIN AGE?

My intention in examining Frenchwomen of a certain age is not to denigrate the rest of us. But after years of close scrutiny with an intellectually honest eye, I am forced to admit that very often, they look better than the rest of us do.

Let me clarify. They don't always look younger, but they definitely tend to present themselves in more chic, more soignée, and more polished packages that can make them *appear* younger. Furthermore, they seem to pull this off with the greatest of ease, while deriving sensual pleasure from every gesture.

Radiant self-confidence is a big part of Frenchwomen's success. But perhaps what many of us don't realize is that pragmatism is also a crucial factor. Frenchwomen of a certain age are realists; realism is at the heart of all of their choices and actions. They accept that life is unpredictable, which makes it rife with both possibility and peril. It's best to be prepared at all times, inside and out.

Their pragmatic nature makes them resilient on the one hand and flexible on the other. Growing older is not without obstacles, but Frenchwomen *expect* obstacles. Happily ever after does not exist in the real world, but beauty, substance, joy, culture, and the ability to accommodate and accept these realities can make for a rich, fulfilling life.

Frenchwomen appreciate the beauty of simplicity, and they understand that the essence of luxury is always quality over quantity. They have constructed their unique styles with a critical eye toward what works *specifically* for their personalities, their bodies, and their best features, and as the decades pass, they adjust and polish their images into nonchalant, uniquely personal expressions of timeless elegance.

I often think back to an interview I conducted many years ago with the director of the Musée des Arts Decoratifs. I asked him why French culture is so universally revered. He maintained that the inherent elegance and style that permeate most aspects of French life can be easily explained as the "natural result of centuries of everyday exposure to beauty in everything from architecture and objects to clothes and food."

An almost unconscious cultural absorption of the lovely and celebration of the pleasing: I think he was onto something. Frenchwomen of a certain age are the very essence of their rich culture—the standard-bearers of its traditions, elegance, and *art de vivre*. I can attest to the fact that they become more and more fascinating over time, while remaining ever vibrant and alluring— inside and out.

HOW FRENCHWOMEN REDEFINE BEAUTY

With the exception of, say, Catherine Deneuve, few French-women are (or were) great beauties. Look at Inès de la Fressange, for example. She is one of a kind and spectacular. Is she a classic beauty? No, she is not. (And, what does she recommend as the world's most important, ageless beauty secret? A smile. I don't believe I have ever seen a picture of her without one.)

Frenchwomen do not aspire to be anyone other than themselves. Perhaps that at least partly explains their general disregard for age as it applies to beauty. And it stands to reason that a culture that creates its own definition of beauty can and does ignore negative connotations associated with age. Frenchwomen, in my view, have refined and redefined both aging and beauty. Birthdays are of little importance, and beauty is wide open to interpretation, by women and men. Instead of dreading her birthday, a Frenchwoman sees the day as an excuse for a celebration of a life well lived, full of experience and adventure, and perhaps a good reason to go shopping and have a facial before taking her time dressing to perfection for a dinner honoring another *anniversaire*.

When I interviewed Jean-Louis Sebagh, the rock star of French plastic surgeons, who practices in France and London, I asked him whether or not Frenchwomen undergo face-lifts. "Of course they do," he assured me, but he qualified that statement, saying, "They do not want anything obvious. They want natural."

Naturel: Frenchwomen's inevitable approach to just about everything in life, even though the means to the end may involve some unnatural intervention.

In my experience, age is not a French obsession. Frenchwomen simply aspire to look the best they can for their age, and they apply themselves to the task. Some have face-lifts and many—I see them sitting in the waiting room at my dermatologist's office, side by side with major French film stars—have youth-enhancing "tweaks." No one is visiting a dermatologist or a plastic surgeon for a radical, unrecognizable change to her visage. Basically, they like themselves, or they've learned to accept themselves and make the very best of their natural resources.

From my friends, I hear little complaining about the march of time, except in jest. Maybe a brief mention of needing to loosen a notch or two on a favorite belt, or to wear it slung lower (but never to abandon it). Many prefer to take the ultra-natural approach by eating well, which they have done their entire lives, watching the scale, exercising, and generally getting on with life with no help from needles or scalpels. When we are together, we discuss our favorite face creams, whether to cut our hair (or not), the sometimes unpleasant truth about upper arms, the life-changing benefits of kiwis for breakfast... all interspersed with detours into what books we're reading, who saw the latest art exhibition, the new trend in the political primaries, the latest app on flower arranging. They care about style, but also about substance.

Frenchwomen are curious, not necessarily spon-taneous or whimsical, but most definitely informed and lively. This is part of their allure. They have opinions—informed opinions—and love nothing better than a heated, though never aggressive, debate. They are, as you know, great flirts. Harmless coquetry, sparkling exchanges, and charm are their greatest arms. All timeless, all recipes for staying young.

What we sometimes forget—and the media is helping us lose our memories in this regard—is that beauty, style, sensuality, generosity, wit, and charm have no expiration dates. We must learn to believe this and act accordingly, like Frenchwomen of a certain age.

DISCIPLINE WILL SET US FREE

My friends and I, while sipping champagne or tea—depending upon the hour—laugh about how blithely unaware we were that everything was easy when we were younger. Slather on this; drink that. Remember to wear sunscreen. Don't eat another one of those. Okay, one more glass of wine; finish that bottle of water. Go ahead, have a piece of chocolate. Lose a few pounds…

We all agree that the drill remains the same, with a few more imperatives thrown in, but the difficulty factor has amped up as the forces of the elements, our hormones, and life in general throw additional challenges at us. One of the nutritionists I interviewed noted that menopause requires cutting two hundred fifty calories from daily intake just to keep weight stable.

Are Frenchwomen disturbed by such trifles? No, they are not. Okay, so the details become even more important, but that doesn't make getting dressed and getting out there any less fun for them. They've been in training all their lives. Why would they stop now? It all starts with discipline. Discipline is the foundation upon which all the rest is built. Do not think for one instant that "discipline" is a dirty word, or an unsavory concept. It is anything but. Discipline is

The Real

FOUNTAIN OF YOUTH

For several years I've been teaching advanced English conversation classes as part of an adult education program in the town near our village. These classes make me feel even more integrated into French society. My students range in age from forty-four to seventy-five. As you might imagine, they are the perfect subjects for the non-scientific surveys whose results I often post on my blog.

◆

For the purposes of this chapter, I decided to ask them what keeps them young. This is what they told me, in no particular order:

❖ Travel.

❖ Classes in everything from painting and computers to golf and yoga—and English, of course.

❖ Annual museum memberships.

❖ Children and grandchildren.

❖ Entertaining.

❖ Fresh air and long walks.

❖ Eating lots of fruits and vegetables. (A few have *potagers*, as do we; we live in the country, after all.)

❖ Sex.

You'll note, not one mentioned a favorite cream or beauty trick.

liberating. It gives a woman—the fates notwithstanding—complete and absolute control over her life.

Frenchwomen do not see the process of caring for themselves as an onus; it is their pleasure to pamper and primp the exterior while always, always educating and expanding their intellect, their curiosity for life. All very, very French and all very, very attainable. But for us, it seems pulling ourselves together is often considered a daunting burden. We have somehow missed the pleasure factor. Yet, as an American living here and watching my friends and acquaintances, I've learned it can be easy. Really, it can.

THE FUN FACTOR: be honest, don't you feel better after a pedicure, a facial, a great haircut, when you wear divine underpinnings, spritz on your favorite perfume? Frenchwomen understand this intrinsically. Taking care of oneself is what builds the confidence we so admire in Frenchwomen.

You're already asking, "Isn't that going to take a lot of time? Can I handle another obligation in my life?" Well, yes. In the beginning, until you weave your new rituals into your routine and they become habits, you will have to schedule extra minutes here and there. May I suggest that you substitute the word "pleasure" for "obligation" and think of self-pampering as something you deserve? Again, think French.

The rewards are immediate—they truly are. In a month your skin will appear younger, your world's-best-ever haircut will save precious minutes of fussing every day and every week.

Pulling together a workable, elegant wardrobe will dispel time-wasting panic attacks and, as a result, bring you new self-assurance.

Frenchwomen eat well, drink little, and take the time necessary to perform their serious daily *toilette*, the ritual ablutions of skin, hair, and body care. Their skin maintenance regimes are not annoyingly necessary chores any more than blithely (and lightly) applying makeup each morning is. These daily ministrations are essential, constructive gestures that start the day on a positive note. They are a woman's investment in herself, the best investment she can make—the one that keeps paying dividends.

REMEMBER, NO ONE IS INVISIBLE

The first step is the decision: Yes, I'm busy. My life is overwhelming. I have exceedingly important things to accomplish; frankly, it never ends. Fine. In a harried, complicated life, when the desire is there to pull back and evaluate one's natural resources, the time can be found. Like a Frenchwoman, I've learned to make myself a priority. This is not selfish; it's intelligent.

No Frenchwoman ever thinks, "I'll just run to the store in this sloppy old sweatshirt and flip-flops and no makeup." She understands that she is not invisible, and she doesn't care if she doesn't see anyone she knows. She has too much self-respect and self-esteem to be unconcerned with her appearance. I know a woman who actually said that she wouldn't answer the door to the water-meter man if she hadn't finished her makeup. "He'll come back," she said.

As Coco Chanel said, "I don't understand how a woman can leave the house without fixing herself up a little—if only out of politeness. And then, you never know, maybe that's the day she has a date with destiny. And it's best to be as pretty as possible for destiny." Indeed.

While we're on the subject of fabricating a seemingly flawless façade, no Frenchwoman in her right mind would ask her husband or companion if he thought she had a large derriere or if he noticed she had gained weight. As my best French friend, Anne-Françoise, said, "Why would you point out anything negative, particlarly if no one has noticed? It's insane, *non*?

"When I was young, I ran around in front of my husband in a pair of tiny bikini panties and a flimsy, filmy silk bra, because everything was perfectly toned," she told me. "Now, even though I'm slim, six children and many years later, everything is not as perky as it once was. I certainly have no intention of pointing this out to my husband. These days it's the packaging that has changed: silk camisole, tap pants, open, flowing kimono, and—because I have good

> "*I don't understand how a woman can leave the house without fixing herself up a little—if only out of politeness. And then, you never know, maybe that's the day she has a date with destiny. And it's best to be as pretty as possible for destiny.*"
> —Coco Chanel

legs—mules with kitten heels to give me a little lift. He thinks I'm just changing the routine. Tell me why any woman with half a brain would want the man in her life to think she was hiding something unattractive?"

A Frenchwoman knows her strengths, conceals her weaknesses, and almost never—except with her closest friend—talks about her fears, failures, or flaws. We Americans have a tendency to tell everyone everything too quickly in a relationship, perhaps in an attempt to be liked. And sometimes we come to regret our indiscretion, our lack of discipline. Frenchwomen are not overly concerned with being liked, and they know a soupçon of mystery is magic.

THE MAGIC EQUATION:
EFFORT + DISCIPLINE = MAJOR REWARDS

I think if someone were to ask me, "What is the single most important lesson you have learned from your friendships with and observations of Frenchwomen?" I would answer, "The smallest effort has major rewards, everything from setting a dining table with care—every day—to getting up, getting dressed, and getting out there to see what adventures the new day holds."

My friend Anne-Françoise, mother of six, grandmother of twelve, interior decorator, hostess extraordinaire, mistress of two large homes, told me she is lazy, which is why she is organized. "I could never accomplish anything if I lived in chaos," she said.

Sometimes I open her linen closets and kitchen cabinets for inspiration. Everything is arranged, not only logically, but also beautifully: pretty papers on shelves, lavender sachets snuggled among her crisply ironed linen sheets—the same ones her grandmother had, she's had for ages, still in pristine condition.

"Yes, I'm well organized and I suppose that means I'm disciplined, but to me that's the only way not to waste time I can use for more pleasurable pursuits," she explained. "I prefer to enjoy my time reading, or having a facial, or drinking tea and gossiping with you, for example."

Anne-Françoise is not a maniac in this respect. She is not a pillow-plumper, as I call those who rush to slap the cushions on their sofa the second a seat is vacated. She makes everything appear effortless, from her dinner parties to her dressing and grooming.

She is able to accomplish these feats because backstage, all the props are in position.

She can still slide into most of the clothes she wore back in the day; those well-tended linens that have lasted so long are the rule, not the exception. The same holds true for her wardrobe. She told me, "I take very good care of my clothes. I respect them because they make me look and feel good and some were very expensive. The pieces from the 1960s and 1970s that are just too young for me—I want to look young, but not ridiculous—I've given to my daughters, but my shirtwaist dresses, skirts, and some jackets and dresses I've been wearing for more than thirty years. Obviously, even though I've tried to keep my weight relatively stable, my body has changed, and that's where my seamstress comes in, or I simply wear my clothes in a different way. If I can no longer button my shirtdress at the waist, it can turn into a lightweight coat to wear over a T-shirt and jeans."

I saw her do this with a pale blue denim shirtdress, and it looked terrific.

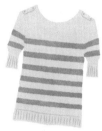

A Frenchwoman's discipline extends far beyond the material. It is one of the guiding principles of her existence and part of the legacy she inherited and will pass on to her own children. And no, discipline does not preclude the occasional flight of fancy. Even the most disciplined Frenchwoman wanders off course from time to time. It's part of enjoying life to the fullest. Remember that other famous French expression, *joie de vivre*? How could one possibly have joy in her life if she didn't allow herself chocolate cake and champagne? *Exactement.*

AGE BEFORE BEAUTY

At a recent dinner with friends, Marechal, the host, and I were talking about age, beauty, charm, Socrates (I swear), sex, politics—the standard conversational topics explored *à table* at a typical French party—and he remarked that he would much rather be seated next to an elegant, lively, fascinating eighty-year-old woman than a gorgeous twenty-five-year-old who had nothing to say.

"I want to enjoy a woman, hear about her experiences, see the sparkle in her eyes," he said. "A vapid young beauty bores me. This age thing, I don't get it. Age literally has no importance."

Ten Secrets to
REMAINING FOREVER CHIC

⌒⌒⌒⌒

Since we all love a how-to guide, *n'est-çe pas*, these ten rules guarantee intangible but noticeable results: you will look younger and more stylish and, as a result, you'll feel more confident. That, in turn, will make you look even better. It's a never-ending cycle.

1. POSTURE. Head held high, shoulders back at all times—when standing, walking, or sitting. (The body adjusts into a perfect line, clothes look better, the effect is physically and psychologically magical. You'll see.)

2. ENOUGH ALREADY. Natural is your aesthetic *raison d'être*. Minimal makeup, hair that moves when you do, nothing fussy or fixed that will detract from an air of nonchalance. (That also applies to clothes and accessories—anything too stiff or constricting automatically looks uptight and dowdy.)

3. MAINTENANCE. Budget time and money for personal upkeep. You're worth it. You are your own best investment. No one knows this better than Frenchwomen of a certain age. (Remember: this is an investment tip, not a guilt-trip. You *owe* it to yourself.)

4. GET OVER IT. Learn to turn what you don't like into an asset. Move on. Don't obsess. We're grown-ups now and worrying about trifles only leads to wrinkles.

5. YOU ARE UNIQUE. Accentuate the positive. There are no negatives, only differences. Different means individual, one of a kind. That's you.

6. EVERY DAY IS AN OCCASION. Frenchwomen live by this rule. Get up, get dressed, and get out there. You owe it to yourself, your self-esteem, and your audience—whether you know the members of that audience or not. (The rewards will abound, you'll see.)

7. BE KIND. Always be gracious and polite. This applies to your interactions with everyone—family, friends, and strangers. Cliché or not, a smile *is* the world's best face-lift. And no, I don't find Frenchwomen parsimonious with their smiles, particularly now that they've caught on to the very American beauty secret of whitening their teeth.

8. *POÉSIE* IN MOTION. Lope, saunter with purpose, put a bounce in your step. Move with grace and energy. There's no need to strut in stilettos; ballet flats work just as well and look every bit as chic and young—if not more so.

9. FLOAT ON A CLOUD—OF FRAGRANCE. Never forget a spritz or a splash. It will be appreciated near and far. Perfume is not a special-occasion indulgence; it is an extension of one's personality.

10. FAKE IT 'TIL YOU MAKE IT. How confident is anyone really? Who knows? Apply all of the above and you will *appear* vibrant and confident. That's the ultimate youth and beauty trick. (Tried, tested, and approved by *moi*.)

My-Reason-For-Living-In-France immediately chimed in his agreement. (Well, I *was* sitting across the table from him.)

Over time, the French have invented monikers for women who shimmer with a magic quite apart from the "norms" one often applies to age and beauty. *La beauté du diable* (the beauty of the devil), for example, was always used to describe the allure of Brigitte Bardot. The expression indicates a beauty that is so sparkling, it will quickly burn out—a beauty of youth, and then *whoosh*, it's gone.

There are also the *jolies laides* (the pretty/ugly women) like the famous socialite Jacqueline de Ribes. Édith Piaf, Colette, George Sand, Charlotte Gainsbourg, and her half-sister Lou Doillon are just some of the many, many women who fall into this category. Most would no doubt include Coco Chanel in the lineup. These women are far more interesting, looking than those whose features meet society's standard definition of beauty.

Each has created herself (and continues to do so in the case of Gainsbourg and Doillon) in her own image. Not one ever tried to squeeze into a mold of youth or beauty. They all share a comfort in their own skin, physically and psychologically.

These women have shaped their singular definition of beauty. There is a marvelous French word that applies here: *bluffant*. *Bluffant* literally means "bluffing," but it has a positive connotation and is also used to mean "mystifying" or "amazing" or "impressive." This perfectly describes the *jolies laides*. They are remarkably original in their style. Adjectives like *jolies* and *belles* are often used to describe them, but they are far more interesting to observe than the everyday banal "pretty" women who carelessly, and wrongly, believe pretty looks are all the ammunition a woman needs. Not true, and French girls and women understand this at their core.

Frenchwomen of a certain age know what works for them, from their hair to their wardrobes and beyond, and as a result, they look fresh and soignée throughout their lives. They cast a spell that makes us redefine outmoded notions of youth and beauty. The confidence they project alone makes them irresistible, ageless.

With conviction, perseverance, and practice, anyone can acquire confidence. It's true, discipline is required, but discipline soon morphs into habit, and the habit is addictive, I can assure you. First you must *believe* you are exceptional, youthful, stunning, and interesting. Emphasize the positive; if you don't believe there are no negatives, *pretend* you believe. With time, confidence will reign.

Confidence is constructed over time, and Frenchwomen of a certain age long ago built the foundation; they polish their images daily. They firmly defined their styles and figured out what works for their figures and lifestyles decades ago. Their wardrobes are well constructed and multifunctional. The pieces fall into place without hysteria. Their beauty regimes are simple, but efficacious. They spend serious money on their hair, which they consider an essential investment—thus no bad-hair days, one fewer concern. No accessory or item of clothing goes back into the closet with a stain, a button missing, wrinkles. Details, details, details. Discipline, discipline, discipline.

SHE IS HER OWN TOP PRIORITY

Let me give you a foolproof recipe for building confidence: Practice saying no.

Non is a word every French-woman pronounces with ease, every day. Follow-up excuses and explanations are not required. When a Frenchwoman says no, she is also saying yes to making herself one of her top priorities. Taking care of herself on all fronts keeps her *en forme*—which includes her good humor—for the important things in her life: her husband, her family, her friends, her job, her passions, and looking stylish.

I see life differently after living in France. I have come to appreciate and incorporate certain aspects and habits of the Frenchwomen I admire into my life. They do not regard taking care of themselves as taking care away from others or other responsibilities. There is no contradiction, no conflict of interest. Feeling good is considered healthy, not selfish.

What keeps them young in my eyes are not only their physical aspects—their hair, makeup, clothes, posture, fluid gestures—but also the intellectual endeavors they pursue. The Frenchwomen I know are voracious readers, museum-goers, international film buffs, and conversation masters.

Maybe it's all that magnesium in the mineral water they glug down throughout the day, but whatever the source, the Frenchwomen I know are brimming with energy and enthusiasm. Perhaps that's the true fountain of youth—that, a great haircut, and a perfect little black dress.

Now, chapter by chapter, you'll see exactly how they do what they do so well.

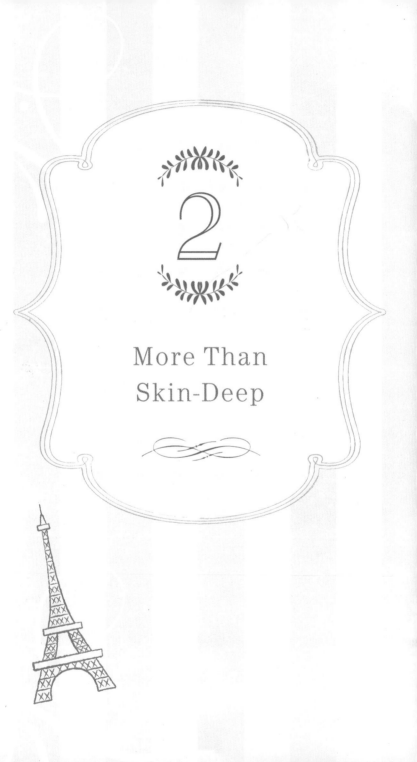

2

More Than
Skin-Deep

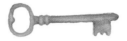

A CELEBRATION OF *LA TOILETTE FRANÇAISE*

Is it culture? Is it nature? Is it nurture? Those were the prevailing questions that danced through my mind when I set out to discover why Frenchwomen of a certain age have complexions that appear completely radiant, yet so natural.

Does culture play a role? *Oui et non*. What about chromosomes? Ah, *non*.

Genetics play no greater role in their appearance than they do in ours. However, *inheritance* is primordial. Under the care and counsel of their mothers and grandmothers, French girls inherit good habits, the primary explanation of the fact that Frenchwomen of a certain age have glowing, youthful looking skin throughout their lives.

Let me assure you, though, before we continue: it is *never* too late to begin taking special care of your face and body. Measurable, radiant results will be your reward. I promise. Although I've taken good care of my face over the years (thanks to my mother), with the advice I've accumulated from French dermatologists, internists, estheticians, plastic surgeons, pharmacists, and friends, I have seen a remarkable improvement in what the French call the *éclat,* or sparkle (*éclat* is a surface that reflects light), and texture of my skin.

In this chapter, I will tell you—from face to feet, detail by detail, ritual by ritual, secret by secret—everything I've learned about how Frenchwomen approach the care and maintenance of their skin and, once again, how they take pleasure in the process.

HOW FRENCHWOMEN PROTECT
THEIR NATURAL RESOURCES

Everyone agrees, a woman's skin does not necessarily coincide with her chronological age and, yes, it can be younger looking than she actually is. The notion never occurred to me, but now it seems persuasively obvious.

Of course, Frenchwomen treat their faces with the greatest care and delicacy, but not one millimeter of their skin is neglected. Just because under ordinary circumstances one can't see every inch doesn't mean it shouldn't be pampered. Daily, creams and lotions follow showers, baths, and the rinse-off after hours in a pool or the ocean. Rich oils and butters (more on this in a second) are applied as intensive treatments to hydrate the body, particularly after a long winter undercover. And both the unseen and the face are treated ever so gently. For example, if you like the effect of a good scrub with ramie or sisal bath gloves, boil the gloves first. Yes, that's right. Pascale, director of the friendly, neighborhood Bernard Cassière spa in the four-teenth arrondissement, says they are too abrasive in their natural state. She likes them once they've been cooked for a couple of minutes. (You'll see. The difference is remarkable, and the exfoliating benefits are equally effective.)

Care and maintenance rituals, I'm convinced, depend partially on a woman's personality—combined with time constraints and discipline. Some of us bask in the joy of a lengthy *toilette*, the ceremony of bathing and grooming. Others of us have neither the leisure nor the inclination to indulge in a drawn-out process. But either way, pleasure should be part of the procedure. Why do some women see beauty ministrations as a chore?

Frenchwomen do not.

I think the idea requires a rethink for us. Think French. Take joy where you find it; create it where you can. Believe me, taking good care of one's self, starting from the top, is the gift to yourself that keeps on giving.

I have tested every product and process I tell you about, and I can assure you that after applying the advice in these pages, you, too, will appear younger, need less makeup, and spend more time accepting compliments than you do performing your new beauty routines.

FRENCHWOMEN LOVE THEIR DERMATOLOGISTS

Perhaps one of the most valuable lessons I've learned from my French friends is that every woman must have her very own dermatologist. I have to admit, this was a surprise for me, as I had never been to a dermatologist except with my mother, who had serious skin allergies. (Her doctor was Austrian and way back then he told my mother to keep me out of the sun as much as possible and to use a sunblock he prescribed. Luckily for me, long before sun worshipping was found to be one of our worst enemies, I was being protected.)

According to doctors and estheticians, the licensed skin specialists who perform facials, hair removal, various beauty-related body treatments—you know, all those treatments that make us want to check into a spa—self-diagnosis is the single major mistake a woman can make when caring for her skin. Carole Doubilet, esthetician and director of the smart Sothys spa in Paris, told me, "A woman may think her skin is dry or oily, for example, but those sensations could merely be a reaction to the wrong products or exceptional exposure to the elements, including heat and air-conditioning."

Though estheticians and dermatologists don't always agree on everything, on that subject there are no arguments. Most women choose cleansing and treatment products by relying upon random recommendations from friends, advertisements, sales personnel, and editorial spreads in their favorite magazines. We compile information, but it may have no relevance for us. "It's a waste of time, effort, and money," Doubilet points out. "A professional can examine a woman's face and tell her exactly the condition of her skin. From that moment forward, she will know how to take care of it properly."

Dermatologists are members of Frenchwomen's indispensable coteries, and as time marches on, relationships with them become ever more intimate and indispensable. Of course, a dermatologist is there for problems, but from my experience, she also comes as close as one can to providing a prescription for the fountain of youth without general anesthesia. Valérie Gallais, a prominent Paris dermatologist who has movie-star clients (I've seen them slink down the hallway into her office), told me that unless a woman has a serious skin condition requiring medical treatment, she advises her patients to schedule annual visits.

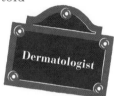

"I do a classic head-to-toe examination, looking for melanomas or other spots that may draw my attention. After, we sit down and discuss beauty," she said. "It's more fun for a woman to conclude an appointment on an upbeat note. In my diagnostic exam I also assess the condition of her face. I ask new patients about their lifestyles, products, and beauty routines. If they're using the wrong products for their skin, I'll explain, or if they can tolerate a more potent formula—and they would see more dramatic results—I will recommend another product or give them a prescription for something more *performant*," meaning something that works better, produces more remarkable results.

"Often, patients who have been coming to me for years need to change brands or move on to stronger versions in the same line because their skin has changed. Formulations must evolve with a woman. It's probable she shouldn't be using the same cream at fifty she used at forty or forty-five. Even five years may be too long to stay loyal to a specific product; it might be necessary to bump it up a notch or two."

LET'S BE PERFECTLY CLEAR: A dermatologist is *not* a luxury. A dermatologist is our greatest anti-aging ally, translation: a necessity. It's possible to find a good dermatologist with whom one can develop a relationship no matter where we live. A yearly checkup with her, as with a gynecologist, is often covered by insurance. No one will call the police if you talk about anti-aging creams and moisturizing masks for a few minutes.

Dermatologists are an investment with major payoffs. If we follow the simple rules they proffer for care and cleansing, we will need practically no makeup and the makeup we do wear will appear invisible—completely *naturel*, exactly like that worn by a Frenchwoman of a certain age.

I've also discovered the products they recommend over the counter, and the more serious products for which they write up prescriptions, are a fraction of the price of less potent and far less effective brands in display-worthy packaging with mega advertising revenues behind them. So the investment pays off in your pocketbook as well. Remember, taking care of ourselves is not an indulgence. It is a requirement for our well-being and, as a consequence, the well-being of those we love. Maintenance can accommodate any budget.

THE BATTLE AGAINST TIME:
ANTI-AGING PRODUCTS

Anti-aging products should begin to be introduced into a woman's beauty regime when she is thirty, the professionals emphasize. Since this information was irrelevant for me, I rushed out and bought my daughter all the products Dr. Gallais recommended and sent them off to Chicago.

The minimum necessities, according to Dr. Gallais, include the magic threesome: a cleansing product and two moisturizing creams or lotions—one for day, plus a richer formula for night (you knew that). In these hydrating products, the age-defying ingredients will give an extra boost to efficaciousness. Keep in mind that they must be chosen specifically for one's skin type, age, and/or any special problems (in all cases, that's where a professional keeps us on message)

Hydrate, hydrate, hydrate is the mantra of all skin professionals, and to make life less complicated, they agree, look for sun protection in the formula of a day cream.

DR. GALLAIS'S GENERAL ADVICE: "All moisturizing products depend upon one's age. Generally, vitamin C is the first step into anti-aging for young women; hyaluronic acid, vitamin A, and glycolic acid are more appropriate for mature skin. Although I often recommend a retinoid product [such as Retin-A] for younger women."

In the United States, it's interesting to note, glycolic acid is often recommended for twenty- and thirtysomethings for both acne control and its anti-aging benefits.

It's important to start slowly. Dermatologists caution that a woman should gradually increase the strength of her anti-aging products—start light and move up the scale as the skin demands. Too much is too much. As with any prescription, no benefit is accrued by overtreating a problem. "Make your skin work," they advise. "Don't give it too much too soon. It's counterproductive," Dr. Gallais said. As our skin evolves, the idea is for us to evolve with it, helping it along without giving it more support than it needs. Dermatologists and estheticians are in accord on this. The skin should "perform" for its reward. At forty, for example, a woman's skin probably does not need an ultra-rich hydrating product, but at sixty it very well might. Products should evolve with a woman, taking into account hormonal changes.

Jean-Louis Sebagh, one of the world's most famous plastic surgeons, is a huge believer in maintenance to slow down the passing of time. He agrees about starting young, in one's thirties, and believes tweaks of Botox, fillers, peels, and laser treatments should also be part of a youth-protecting program. "Not a lot, just enough," he said. "Remember, French women do not like anyone to think they're doing anything 'unnatural,' which means as they keep up the maintenance, no one sees radical changes and therefore no one notices. It all *appears* natural."

He calls these procedures "fine tunings." Sebagh says he doesn't "change faces," but rather helps restore them. "You can keep your forty-year-old face until you're seventy if you start early with medical maintenance." The medical maintenance to which he is referring can include a cocktail of laser treatments, Botox, hyaluronic fillers, mesotheraphy (more on this in a moment), and injections (antioxidant vitamins C, A, and E), all administered in the hands of a highly qualified doctor, preferably one who, like Dr. Sebagh, has an artist's sensibility. He claims that these minimally invasive procedures can perform miracles.

So, I asked Dr. Sebagh, what the minimum investment would be for the miracle of keeping a forty-year-old face until one is seventy.

"That's such an American question," he said.

"Perhaps, but please humor me," I said.

"About 2,500 euros a year," he said, "but I have some patients who spend upwards of 10,000."

Most of us, for various reasons—philosophy, budget, fear—prefer a softer approach to our beauty regimens, which means we must rely on good sense, good food, trusted dermatologists, and good products. Good fortune, as in good genetics, never hurts either, but that's the luck of the draw.

For several years I was using a vitamin C serum and its complementary cream, both recommended by Sandrine Sebban, an internist who is one of France's leading doctors of aesthetic medicine. Vitamin C is an antioxidant that "traps" free radicals that accelerate the aging process. Serums and creams with a base ingredient of vitamin C improve the skin's density, resulting in fewer signs of age. Dr. Gallais told me so.

Free radicals age skin by increasing destruction of collagen, the fiber that keeps skin flexible and smooth. Vitamin C is highly effective for maintaining collagen, but it is itself unstable. The only form of vitamin C that remains effective is L-ascorbic acid, which must be kept in a dark, light-shielding bottle. (My Flavo-C serum is sold in such a bottle, and Dr. Sebban also told me to store my bottle inside my medicine chest to ensure further protection.)

It's comforting to know there is serious science behind a product, but all I care about are results. Vitamin C is suitable for all skin types and, yes, I've seen a measurable difference. My skin appears almost poreless and baby smooth—air kissers have complimented me on my smooth cheeks—and it has a youthful rosy, glow. I need very little makeup.

My prescription Retin-A, which my skin tolerates well, although that is not the case for some women, has been one of my greatest allies for more than twenty years. As a result of nightly—yes, perhaps excessive—use, I have no upper lip "bar code" lines, nor do I have the classic lion's whatchamacallit between my brows.

Dr. Sebagh said, "There is no question that these products are one of the most remarkable anti-aging solutions that have ever existed. They are part of our toolbox. Prevention is always the best medicine."

If you can tolerate Retin-A, I recommend requesting a prescription. It's another never-too-late remedy. If you have redness and flaking side effects, Dr. Gallais suggests NeoStrata Renewal as an alternative. To treat redness and flaking, Anti-Rougeurs Nuit, a rich cream from Eucerin, solves the problem, she said.

Unfortunately, it never occurred to me to apply my Retin-A to my nasolabial folds, those nasty parentheses between the nose and lips. Somehow I don't think it would have made that much difference. One esthetician remarked that I must have smiled a lot in my life. How true.

ANOTHER HARD TRUTH: Retin-A was not created to fill in the creases in those areas where our faces have lost volume. That's where fillers come in. And, as you know, fillers come in syringes.

But never mind, since Dr. Sebagh told me that smiling is the best facial exercise that exists, I couldn't be happier. "Smiles are 'elevators,' grimaces and frowns are 'depressors,' and then there is gravity, so it's best to elevate as much as possible," he said.

Serious anti-aging products can and should be used on the *décolleté*. This often forgotten area can let us down sooner than we think. Unfortunately, I was careless on that front and had the crinkles to prove it. We often blithely slather creams, lotions, and SPF products on our faces but forget our delicate neck and chest areas. To deal with my carelessness after the fact, I first turned to my trusty Retin-A to see if it could remove some of the damage. It didn't. The results were disappointing at best. Then I turned to Dr. Gallais and the magic of mesotheraphy.

You can't get much more French than mesotherapy. Frenchwomen adore mesotheraphy. They refer to it as an aesthetic anti-aging treatment—or, more likely, they don't refer to it at all.

Mesotherapy was developed by a French doctor, Michel Pistor, in 1952, and in 1987, it was recognized by the French National Academy of Medicine as an integral part of traditional medicine. But Dr. Gallais was not using the procedure on my chest (or on her patients generally) under the umbrella of traditional medicine. Her intervention was strictly cosmetic.

Mesotheraphy is a minimally invasive procedure that targets problem areas. It has multiple beauty-related uses—plumping hands and reducing crow's-feet, for example—and is performed with micro-injections of, in my case, a cocktail of vitamins and hyaluronic acid. Yes, a needle is involved, but it is only about a quarter of an inch long and extremely fine. "Isn't it cute?" Dr. Gallais asked rhetorically as she brandished it for me to see. (This is the point where she gently wiped off the *verrrrry* thick anesthetic cream I had applied before the appointment.)

Tiny "medical bullets" are delivered directly into the middle layer of the skin, the mesoderm. The technique is a *nappage* (think dot, dot, dot, dot…) of the wrinkled area. Truly, it's no pain, all gain. The number of treatments one needs varies, of course. I was content after two at eighty euros each. The cocktail delivered by syringe stimulates natural collagen and elastin, and therefore the process is "natural," with a little help from the medical community. Hyaluronic acid injected beneath the skin has the potential to capture thirty times its size and volume in water, which leads to formation of polymers that hydrate and add volume to the skin. At the same time, it helps repair the skin because it boosts new cell production and microcirculation.

To keep up the good work, typically the procedure should be repeated annually. I couldn't be happier with the results and plan on adding this to my beauty to-do list. At the same time, I shall never again forget to hydrate below my neck or neglect a proper SPF product. Live and learn.

An appointment with Joëlle Ciocco, hailed in French *Vogue* as "the world's most famous epidermitologist" ("epidermitologist" being a word she apparently invented), resulted in a few more products being added to my repertoire. Madame Ciocco is a biochemist and, according to several women I interviewed, a miracle worker. Personally, she exceeds my budget. One of her almost two-hour facials, which she says should probably be done four times a year, takes a neat 1100 euros per facial out of a beauty budget—and she is only putting creams and liquids *on* the face, albeit with masterful movements. Masterful but not always pleasant: at one point she donned a pair of surgical gloves and put her thumbs inside my mouth, with the rest of her hands over the cheeks extending back to my ears. Then she started massaging. She warned me it might be "uncomfortable." Since her hands were in my mouth, I had two choices: bite her—which I seriously considered—or just let the tears roll down my cheeks in silence. Since she only charged me half price, I decided not to cause a scene.

Judging from women of a certain age (and beyond) I've seen who are loyal clients, including international film

A *PETIT* TIP:

Toting your skin care products to your next appointment gives your dermatologist immediate information about your beauty habits.

stars, she seems to produce remarkable results. She also has a huge and expensive product line, but to her great credit, she did not mention one of her potions when she gave me a suggested shopping list of items I should begin using immediately. A brilliant cleanser, Purete Thermale 3-in-1 from Vichy, was at the top of her list.

Another of her recommendations was selenium in ampoule form, which I applied directly to my face, as she advised, three nights a week until I finished the box. Reputedly, selenium increases the action of antioxidants and is a terrific anti-aging tool. Because it seemed odd to me to put it *on* my face, I asked my doctor and my dermatologist what they thought. Both told me the molecules were too large to penetrate the skin, but said selenium is an excellent internal antioxidant, adding that if I enjoyed splitting open the glass ampoules and putting the mineral on my face as a sort of astringent, go ahead and do it, but if I wanted to do something serious for my skin, I should drink the stuff. I started drinking the stuff. Did it change my life? No, but generally speaking, my skin looks great for my age, and I'm assuming everything I do helps.

Selenium can be found naturally in garlic, whole grains, seafood, tuna, eggs, and Brazil nuts, among other foods. Why not work inside and outside? That's always my philosophy.

Dr. Gallais prescribed two supplements for me, which I take daily: Cledist, a compound that includes the magical selenium, plus zinc, vitamin E, vitamin C, and lots of other natural ingredients, including extracts of tomato, blueberry, and grape, along with turmeric, followed by Elteans, which gives me the famous omega-three and omega-six wonders and extracts of soy and carrots. When my liquid selenium ran out, I decided to take only Dr. Gallais's supplements, which I plan to pop for the rest of my life.

INSIDE OUT

Believe it or not, great skin is not just about what we put on our skin or what we avoid. Frenchwomen have learned that what you eat and what you take can have marked impact.

It might be a no-brainer, but everyone told me that one of the worst things we can do to our faces after a certain age is to be a yo-yo dieter. That sort of depressed me since, regrettably, that's the story of my life. At the same time, they emphasized the importance of eating foods that keep us young. YOU KNOW THE DRILL: lots of grains, good protein, and broccoli, for example.

At least one part of us needs some fat—our faces. Apparently, the famous French "ten years on the face for ten pounds on the derriere" maxim is true. I have a couple of friends, though, who would rather keep the derrieres they had at thirty and do the best they can with their faces.

"It's the fat in the face that makes us appear young," Dr. Sebagh said. "It's not the same fat as in the rest of our body; it's more fragile. When we lose mass in the face, we look gaunt. Lack of volume means we look older."

Water. One-and-a-half liters per day is the minimum. Internist Alexandra Fourcade, fifty-one, has her water bottle on her desk in her office. She says some days she refills it three times. Mine is beside me as I write this. Sometimes I put half of a five hundred–milligram effervescent vitamin C tablet into the bottle or spike it with green tea. Vitamin C is an antioxidant. Every little bit helps. Green tea also helps the water go down, with added benefits. Dr. Fourcade approves.

A glass of pomegranate juice in the morning provides a blast of antioxidants. Dr. Fourcade drinks it every day.

Many of us are not always as conscientious or consistent about our five daily servings of fruits and vegetables as we should be. Dr. Gallais and Dr. Sebban, in this case, suggest their patients take a semiannual "cure" of vitamins and antioxidants in capsule form. Both do this themselves. Each cure lasts three months, with a three-month break in between. Of course, I followed my leaders with Oléage Selenium-ACE Progress 50. It contains extracts from grape seed, olives, and tomatoes, known for their antioxidant benefits. Then the makers throw in some broccoli.

WHY DO YOU THINK SHE WAS CALLED "SLEEPING" BEAUTY?

We must have sleep. Our lives may be filled with problems and stress. They sap not only our strength—physical and mental—but also our youth and beauty. Sleep rejuvenates not only the soul, but also the body. If you suffer from insomnia, try herbal pills (mine, recommended by my friend and pharmacist, are a mélange of *Valeriana officinalis*, *Passiflora incarnata*, *Crataegus* sp., and *Ballota nigra* L.), essential oils, or herbal teas. My pharmacist friend Christine Salort also recommended placing three drops of *camomille noble, verveine citronnée,* or *neroli* on a tiny cube of sugar (trust me, you need the sugar) and swallowing it.

Dr. Sebagh also emphasized the importance of sleep for beautiful skin. He never gets fewer than seven hours. He also said we should find ways, whether through meditation or sports, to reduce stress in our lives. "Stress has a biological effect," he said. When stressed, our adrenal glands become overactive and this overactivity is aging.

INSIDE AND OUT: FRENCHWOMEN'S SEASONAL SECRETS

One month before intense exposure to the sun, on a beach or ski vacation, for instance, doctors and pharmacists recommend we prepare our skin for the assault with pre-sun pills. Since I definitely did not understand this extremely popular practice in France, I turned to my pros.

The capsules contain carotenoids, notably lycopene, which accelerates the production of melanocytes to prepare the skin for the sun. The treatment is particularly useful for those who are allergic to the sun, Dr. Gallais explained. Some individuals react to the sun with redness and bumps; preparation with the pre-*soleil* pills helps build up melatonin as a protective barrier against the sun's rays.

The Mayo Clinic defines sun allergy as "a condition in which sunlight triggers a skin reaction. For most people, sun allergy symptoms include an itchy red rash in areas that have been exposed to sunlight. A severe allergy may cause hives, blisters, or other symptoms."

Before buying pre-sun pills, however, it's important to check with your internist or dermatologist to be certain the ingredients are pure and natural. For women of color, these capsules may increase uneven patches of dark color, known as melasma.

The primary ingredients in the capsules we use are tomato lycopene, natural carotenes, selenium (oh, look, selenium again!), and vitamin E.

My friend Sophie, who's forty-seven, has exquisite, creamy white skin, and is allergic to the sun. She starts taking her pills one month before her summer and winter vacations, even though she never intentionally tries to tan.

The pills are a twofer, and we all know how much we love to double our pleasure. They also help us achieve a golden tan while hydrating the skin. They assist in the process of achieving that French *bronzage* look we so admire while at the same time protecting us inside and out. **NEED I ADD:** The treatment does *not* preclude the need for a serious SPF product.

The treatment gives my too-pale skin the slightest hint of color. Since I never intentionally tan either, the result has been a pleasant surprise.

If you're planning to do fillers, Botox, or a more radical intervention, do *not* forget your *Arnica montana* one week in advance and one week after to reduce or, if you're lucky, prevent bruising. When I fell on my face in our driveway, Christine Salort, my pharmacist friend, gave me some immediately. Had I anticipated the serious slip, I would have prepared in advance.

The usual dosage of this homeopathic medication is five pellets, three times daily. Arnica is a member of the daisy family and has been used for centuries, first to relieve indigestion and later to minimize bruising.

SMALL INVESTMENTS, MAJOR RETURNS

"Buy less, invest more" is the motto of every Frenchwoman of a certain age. The credo applies to all aspects of her life. Frugal by nature, Frenchwomen waste neither time nor money.

The doctors I interviewed—whose patients include princesses, countesses, film stars, writers, television personalities, and Frenchwomen of a certain age who want to invest in their futures—told me they love the simplicity and purity of a select few products formulated for babies.

Marie Serre, one of France's leading dermatologists, actually took me into her bathroom to show me her can't-live-without products. For cleansing, she is loyal to Bioderma ABCDerm H2O Solution Micellaire. It comes in a one-liter clear plastic pump bottle and costs about ten euros at Monoprix or any pharmacy. It is specifically made for babies. It's mild, effective, kind to the skin, and requires no rinsing. As you might imagine, a bottle now has pride of place in my bathroom as well. It is surprisingly effective for gently removing mascara.

"I use it every day and have for years," Dr. Serre said.

Like me, she always gives her face a final spritz of thermal water before applying her nighttime products. (A large can of water lasts for months.)

Thermal waters, as spring waters are known in France, are nonirritating, partially because of their low calcium content, and aid in "repairing" (the word used by Dr. Gallais) the skin, and they act as anti-inflammatory agents. I keep mine in the refrigerator in the summer and a small purse-size can in my *sac* to spritz when the temperatures rise.

Dr. Serre even showed me her favorite Lotus cotton pads—also created for babies. The maxi-sized pads are four-and-a-quarter inches by three-and-a-half-inches, with aloe vera built in, and are made for both sides to be used. "First, you squirt the Bioderma on the square," Dr. Serre explained, "then you gently cleanse your face. Next, you turn over the square and start again. When your cotton pad is clean, so is your face." I often put a package or two of these pads into gifts I send to the States. They work as top-notch packing materials, and everyone who receives them asks for more.

THE NO, NO, NOS

It's impossible not to mention the obvious, so here goes: no sun-baking, no cigarettes, no rough stuff when using products. Go light on alcohol and cleanse every night before bed—no matter what. No one is too tired to spend sixty seconds or less removing the grime that accumulates daily. Yes, you know these things—we all do—but a chapter on skin cannot be written without a quick review. *N'est-ce pas?* Dr. Gallais listed as her two most egregious pet peeves "inappropriate, overly harsh products that dry the skin and visits to UV tanning salons." She remarked with dismay that she is continually shocked by women who haven't gotten the message about the dangers therein.

You may think most Frenchwomen smoke. From my experience I rarely meet (or see) a woman of a certain age who does. (Unfortunately, I do see a shocking number of teens and young women who do. If only they would listen to their mothers.) I confirmed my observations with our internist, who said he finds among his patients that women between the ages of forty-five and fifty are stopping the habit in record numbers.

Dr. Fourcade, a former "light smoker," told me that wine for her is part of socializing, and she doesn't drink it every day. "I know the research and the therapeutic values of red wine, but I also know I feel better when I have only the occasional glass or two at table, and studies prove alcohol is aging for the skin. Plus, the calories."

Dr. Gallais concurs. "The occasional *coupe de champagne*? *Pourquoi pas*? One must make exceptions for pleasure from time to time, but daily consumption of alcohol is not a good idea for our faces. Grape juice has antioxidants without the alcohol." If you're worried about staining your teeth, opt for white grape juice.

In all the years I have lived in France, never have I seen a Frenchwoman of any age drink a cocktail or any sort of alcohol other than wine and champagne. I have only one friend who smokes. She admits she uses cigarettes as an appetite suppressant and, unfortunately, she was a sun worshipper most of her life. Seen from the back, with her sublime, naturally platinum hair—a mix of white and blonde— and her tight jeans, she could pass for a twenty-five-year-old. When she turns around, she looks almost three times that age.

Interestingly, she never touches alcohol, not even wine. She accepts a glass at table and leaves it full. With the exception of one of my best French friends, I don't think I have ever seen Frenchwomen at dinner parties drink more than one (maybe two) flutes of champagne as an aperitif and one or two small glasses of red wine at table. But, let me add, those days are exceptions. And not once, in all the years I've lived here, have I ever seen a Frenchwoman tipsy.

A LAST WORD ON ALCOHOL: Don't think that only lack of sleep causes dark circles beneath the eyes. So does alcohol. If nothing else, shadows under the eyes make us appear older.

THE PLEASURES AND BENEFITS OF *LA TOILETTE*
Since we're talking head-to-toe beauty in these pages, I thought, before we continue, you might appreciate an organized presentation for quick, easy reference. I always do. Life is complicated enough.

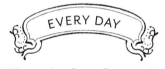

When the Sun Comes Up

- Wash face with a gentle product, rinse with warm water, spray with cool thermal water.
- Oily skin is rare after a certain age, so astringent toners are normally not necessary.
- *Eau de bleuet* (cornflower water) is a completely natural alcohol-free "water" that many French -

women use after cleansing their faces. It also helps close pores.

❖ *Eau de rose* is another secret French water that gives the skin a slight glow—and it smells divine.

❖ Another treat for the senses: the deep blue bottles of *eau de bleuet* and *eau de rose* look beautiful in the bathroom. (Imagine, they were probably used by Marie Antoinette and the Marquise de Pompadour.)

❖ Now comes the day cream. Recently, at the behest of Dr. Gallais, I switched to one with a high hyaluronic acid formula.

NOTE: Hyaluronic acid, a naturally occurring molecule present in our skin, is responsible for the skin's density and retention of water. It is what's in the syringes that fill out those deep lines. Out of a jar, it's considerably less invasive. The molecule is too large to pass through the skin in any external formulations—however, it aids in the penetration of other products, such as vitamins A and C. It has exceptionally potent moisturizing properties and helps plump or, as the French say, "repulp" the epidermis. Ideally, a hyaluronic product should also contain a retinoid, which many experts agree may stimulate the synthesis of collagen and the elasticity of the skin.

❖ To simplify life, at least make sure you have a SPF built into your day cream formula.

❖ The minimum SPF is between 15 and 20 when we're not on an island or at the top of a mountain. Dr. Gallais demonstrated with a graph the enormous disparity between no SPF and 15 to 20 compared to the considerably smaller difference between 20 and 50.

❧ Nothing is not an option.

NOTE: The American Melanoma Foundation and the American Academy of Dermatology recommend a minimum of SPF 30 and urge people to use SPF 50 when engaging in outdoor activities.

❧ I questioned four friends about eye creams. Marie-Claude, Claudine, Marion, and Dany all told me they are fastidious about their creams, but never use specific eye potions. Both my dermatologist and her absolutely gorgeous forty-three-year-old assistant told me they never use eye cream—day or night. See? Another economy.

When the Sun Goes Down

In the evening, *carefully* and *gently* remove every trace of makeup. Rinse and spritz with mineral water again. Some tap water is exceptionally hard, with high concentrations of calcium, which can be drying.

❧ You want a product to remove eye makeup? It's not really necessary. Both my Vichy 3-in-1 creamy cleanser, recommended by Joëlle Ciocco, which I alternate with ABCDerm H2O, the favored choice of Dr. Serre, are champions on even waterproof mascara. The latter is a *micellaire* product, which means no rinsing necessary.

NOTE: Both cleansing products can be found in pharmacies, last for months, and cost just a few euros.

- Now apply vitamin C serum—wait two minutes while it sinks in, then seal it with your night cream. The entire routine takes three-to-four minutes. The results are obvious. The serum/cream combo is not absolutely necessary, but most definitely a good idea.
- Although vitamin C serums can stimulate collagen growth, they are not hydrating, so if you have dry skin, a night cream is an excellent addition.
- If you prefer to skip a step, you can go directly to your specific anti-aging night cream. Remember, skin is all about hydration, hydration, hydration. Since the perfectly clean surface is ready to drink in age-defying products, nighttime is the occasion to use a retinoid and a cream with moisturizing ingredients such as glycerin.
- Remember, our body temperature increases slightly during sleep, which can facilitate deeper absorption of creams and serums.
- Finally, apply a rich body cream.

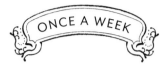

Gommage, or exfoliation, removes dead skin and gives the face an immaculately clean, rosy surface. (I love the word *gommage*; it means "erasure." One uses a *gomme,* or rubber eraser, to erase a word, for example. And it's feminine: *une gomme.*)

- Until recently I thought exfoliation, by definition, removed makeup, but that's not the case, nor the point. Skin must be clean before *gommage*. As Elodie, an esthetician and owner of a trendy spa outside Paris, pointed out, "To exfoliate your face without removing your makeup first is like taking a shower with your clothes on."
- *Gommage* can also be used on slightly chapped lips.
- Follow *gommage* by an appropriate—gentle, always gentle—moisturizing mask. If your skin is particularly oily, which is probably unlikely, ask your dermatologist for a mask that is right for your skin type or follow the exfoliation with your favorite cream.
- As Dominique Rist, international treatment development and training director for Clarins, said, "Skin only understands when you speak gently."
- Often, once we've found the products whose ingredients work for us, the rest of the equation comes down to personal taste. We may like the texture, the aroma, the experience of one over another.

- ❧ **ANOTHER SECRET:** If you leave your moisturizing mask on as a night cream once or twice a week, you'll wake up gorgeous. Tried, tested, true.
- ❧ Moisturizing masks are not goopy. When you have found the one you like best, you'll see that if you wait fifteen-to-twenty minutes before placing your head on your pillow (covered with a fresh, clean pillowcase, of course), you will see beautiful results.

START EARLY!

Experts recommend that a girl should be initiated into the pleasurable practice of proper facial cleansing at age twelve. A mild lotion cleanser is the most fun at that age, and many exist. Using it in place of mundane soap and water is an initiation into the "big girl" world of beauty and, therefore, theoretically, a new, fun experience that will lead to a lifetime of proper skincare habits. If you have any pubescent girls in your family, now is the time to step in and introduce them not only to the products, but also to the enjoyment associated with using them. Dr. Salort, my pharmacist, also noted there are non-soap soaps that offer another alternative before transitioning into more "grown-up" seeming products, noting that most treatment lines have such products in their repertoires—after all, they want to keep girls coming back to them throughout their lives.

If acne is a problem, pharmacists come to the rescue. If the problem persists, a visit to the dermatologist is in order. It's part of the Frenchwoman's mentality: care and treatment foremost, and one is never too young to learn that lesson.

PERSONAL TIPS AND TRICKS
(LEARNED FROM THE EXPERTS, OF COURSE)

Because I truly do enjoy *ma toilette*, I've added a high-tech twist to my routine, which, I might add, has had major payoffs. On my last birthday, I gave myself the gift of a Clarisonic brush. Normally I use it every other night. I'm convinced my follow-up serum and cream work better than ever. I've prepared the terrain, if you will.

My Clarisonic gently (of course) cleanses away the daily accumulation of grime more effectively than manual cleaning. It loosens and whisks away dirt and oil. The brush whirls at three hundred movements per second in order to remove, thoroughly, six times more makeup and two times more oil than cleaning with one's hands alone. (An American friend who is so attached to hers told me, "They will have to pry it out of my cold, dead hand.")

By the time this book is published, the Clarisonic will be sold in France, which it is not at the moment. Some French dermatologists, and Dominique Rist, are against it, believing the device is too harsh and can break delicate capillaries. Therefore, as you can imagine, I took mine with me on a visit to Dr. Gallais. She thought it was wonderful, as long as I put no pressure on it and use the most delicate attachment.

My face feels so, so clean. It has a rosy radiance, and I can tell you, I have seen an appreciable difference in the effectiveness of my beloved products used in combination, i.e., after a Clarisonic deep cleansing.

Because I have sensitive skin, which I only discovered recently, and for the first time ever have had some redness,

Joëlle Ciocco recommended a twice-a-week treatment with a calamine gel, which I didn't previously know existed. I remember calamine lotion from that one time I walked through a patch of poison ivy in the woods next to our house when I was ten, but haven't thought about it since.

Madame Ciocco said it would soothe my skin and cure any inflammation. She told me to use it as a mask and leave it on for fifteen minutes, then rinse and follow with a thermal water spray. I did as I was told. (As you no doubt realize at this point, I'm willing to do almost anything.) Did it work? Maybe. It's soothing. Cause and effect aren't clear.

Finally, a this-is-just-me beauty suggestion. I won't call it a "tip," because when I proposed the idea to the estheticians, I thought they were going to faint. The doctors, however, replied, "Why not?"

Once a week I leave my poor face in peace. I clean it as always, dab my Retin-A in various strategic areas, make sure I have a fresh pillowcase, and go to bed. I let my skin breathe. If it's not an excellent idea, it's not a bad idea, the medical experts agree. Personally, I think it's a splendid idea. When I asked a couple of my French girlfriends what they thought about my "secret," they said they loved it, but didn't think 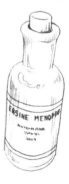 of it in quite the same way. More or less they said that's what they do when they're too tired to do anything more than cleanse.

A HARD TRUTH: when you see advertisements for creams that promise to help restructure and measurably lift the oval—you know, the jawline that has given up the fight with gravity—it's a lie. Three solutions are available: turtleneck sweaters, strategically placed scarves, and, unfortunately, the most effective option, plastic surgery. I know, I know . . . No one ever said life was fair.

THE BODY BEAUTIFUL

Beauty treatments do not stop at the neck. French-women apply the same rigor and discipline to keeping their bodies soft, mostly hair-free, and smelling delicious as they do to tending their faces.

For them, *gommage* and daily moisturizing are golden. You could use your facial exfoliant on your body, but I, and the experts, prefer a more substantial product. The body can handle it, and the results are significantly better.

One of the many benefits of the "investigative reporting" that went into this book were the beauty treatments I scrutinized firsthand. A full-body exfoliation massage feels like you've died and gone to heaven. In a perfect world I would put this on my monthly to-do list.

If you want to make your own, one esthetician suggests a mixture of sweet almond oil and moderately fine sea salt. Sugar works equally well if you think salt is too harsh. Start with a tablespoon of salt (or sugar if you prefer) and mix with the oil until you arrive at a consistency that is pleasing and that works. The French are very much into a dash of this, a handful of that. However, I recommend adding some table salt to your facial exfoliant to turn it into a body *gommage* treatment. (You can break your neck in the shower stepping on slippery oils, and they are extremely difficult to rinse off all surfaces, including the body; that's why I like my recipe.) While working in the crystals, spend extra time on elbows, knees, and heels. Sometimes I use a paste of lemon juice and baking soda on my elbows. I apply it with my pre-boiled exfoliating bath glove in the shower.

On those days when you're rushing about and don't have time for a multistep sloughing, put your body cream on the boiled bath glove and get a light *gommage* followed up with moisturizer when you step out of the shower. That's what Anne-Françoise and Aurore do most of the time.

A daily body moisturizer should have urea as an important component, because urea promotes deep hydration and creates a protective film that seals in moisture. Urea is another molecule naturally present in the skin that fixes water in the epidermis. Products containing 10 percent or more in their formulas erase dry, scaly patches of skin, leaving the surface smooth and elastic. Urea also relieves the itching caused from dry skin. "Use it and it's the end of alligator skin," Dr. Gallais said, showing her arm as proof.

Dr. Gallais recommends a concentration of between 5 and 10 percent, depending upon the condition of one's skin. Again, the richer the better on elbows, knees, heels, and occasionally our hands. If you're looking for glamour, it's not to be found in these creams and lotions, but if you're looking for results, start rubbing.

Emergency TREATMENTS

1) **TOO MUCH CHAMPAGNE?** *Eau de bleuet* (cornflower water) to the rescue. Take several of those flat cotton makeup-remover pads that fit perfectly over the eyes, soak them in eau de bleuet, and put them in the freezer—yes, the freezer. When eyes are puffy and tired, take out a couple, whirl them around in the air so they're not icicles, place them on your eyes, and lie down for three to five minutes. Trust me on this one; it's a mini-homemade miracle.

    Next comes the worst part of the prescription, an icy cold shower. Even one minute under those conditions makes you realize how slowly time passes when you're not having fun. To me, this seems more like a punishment for our excesses.

2) **PUFFY EYES (FOR WHATEVER REASON)?** From my friend Elise, who has solutions for everything (part of this you may know, however, I'm willing to bet you're not familiar with the final detail): steep two chamomile tea bags in boiling water, remove, and place between two cotton pads. Wave in the air until they reach a comfortable temperature. Lie down, put compresses on your eyes, and relax until they become cold. Next, wrap an ice cube in gauze and pass it around the contour of the eyes—five times in one direction, five in the other, slowly and gently.

3) **A TRUE ANTISTRESS TRICK.** Toss two large handfuls of chamomile flowers (you can find them in health food stores) into two quarts of boiling water. Allow to boil for ten minutes and infuse for thirty minutes. Remove the flowers and pour the liquid into your bath. Soak for fifteen minutes. Sipping a cup of green tea or chamomile tea will add to the pleasure.

4) **A REFRESHINGLY PLEASANT PICK-ME-UP.** Pour your *eau de rose* into a small ice cube tray. Take the cubes, covered with gauze, and pass them over the face and neck. It's a lovely experience that closes the pores, and doing the same with a gentle tap-tap-tap motion over makeup helps "fix" the cosmetics.

5) **SOS, MAJOR OCCASION.** You need a little help from a friend. Let me introduce you to mine. On occasion, when I need the big guns, I apply Flavo-C Flash. It's formulated with a protein complex that dries quickly and forms an invisible, flexible—that's important, as you can imagine, that way you can have a conversation and even smile—gel film that provides an instant tightening and smoothing effect. Unfortunately, it has a Cinderella downside. The magic lasts five to six hours only, but while it works, it works. I look rested and fresh and fine lines seem smaller. I do put the Flash around my eyes. But you have to get out of town before the carriage turns into a pumpkin.

6) **YIKES! PIMPLES!** To treat adult acne, Dr. Salort recommends Normaderm from Vichy or Aroma Perfection by Nuxe. She has used both and recommends them to her clients. I didn't test these products for you because, luckily, I've never been plagued with serious acne, only the occasional *bouton*.

When the occasional *bouton* ("button," a much cuter word than "pimple" don't you think?) does appear, I cover it generously with my Retin-A and it usually disappears within two days.

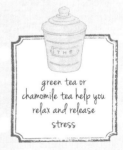

green tea or chamomile tea help you relax and release stress

The above routine is the bare minimum—it works for those who have paid attention to their skin, all their skin, all along. Now let's say there's been some *laissez-aller* ("carelessness"—it wouldn't even occur to me to suggest "laziness") in the area between the neck and feet. Not to worry. Some heavy artillery will save the day.

A super-rich massage butter like shea butter or argan oil, which also exists in a creamy butter form, can make up for our beauty lapses. Both are pure, filled with vitamins, and can be used as deep conditioners for the hair, rubbed into the cuticles, and, of course, massaged over and over on dry areas of the skin until they can no longer absorb any more oil.

I recommend, as do estheticians, that for an intensive, post-pajama winter treatment, we sleep in a layer of the butter. You must have an old pair of sweat bottoms and a T-shirt someplace. Remember your socks. And, do I need to say this? Don't *ever* wear that getup outside the privacy of your own home, and try not to let friends or members of your family see you so attired. Let's not forget this is a book about Frenchwomen.

You might want to do this on the same night you leave your moisturizing mask on your face. And, if you want to go all the way, include your hands, with gloves (of course) and, *pourquoi pas?*, the hair masque I tell you about in the chapter on the subject.

I'm hoping the man in your life will understand that you'll be more beautiful when the mission is accomplished. You can say you're doing it for him—a Frenchwoman would. It makes life *soooo* much easier. Better yet, move into the guest room. You can say you think you might be coming down with a cold and wouldn't want him to catch it . . .

When questioning French friends and acquaintances, I discovered that literally, without exception, every woman had a bottle of argan oil in her beauty arsenal. They use it on their faces, legs, elbows, wherever. Another favorite is sweet almond oil, which some use to remove eye makeup or as a simple, pleasant, no-tech moisturizer. I'm not crazy about the oils for makeup removal, particularly around the eyes, because in my hands, at least, some always seeps into the eyes. Not only is this mildly painful, but oils make the eyes puffy.

A new, at least for me, treatment on offer in some spas in Paris is deep moisturizing with warm, scented beeswax candles. Bernard Cassière sells them with a spout to retrieve the liquid easily. You light the candle, immerse yourself in the soothing perfume, blow the candle out, and wait for the wax to cool from dangerously hot to warm. It is then applied like a cream to the legs, and massaged into dry, scaly skin. I've had heavenly pedicures and manicures using this method in New York but never before had it applied to my legs and arms or rubbed into the skin. Although it works, and the entire experience is divine in the hands of an expert, I would never try this at home. I know it would lead to a major catastrophe that could necessitate medical intervention. Sandrine, an acquaintance, said she would walk from one side of Paris to the other to have one of these treatments. (Normally she drives. She likes to exaggerate.)

Let's get this on and off the table immediately. Cellulite/ drainer products are a great deal of work for difficult-to-measure results.

HERE'S THE THING: for them actually to work, one must vigorously apply them once each day, and for real results, it has been suggested, twice. That's a lot of commitment even for someone who likes her *toilette*. Twice-daily use for the rest of our lives(!). Results promised are smoother skin (read: no visible cellulite), better circulation, less water retention, and a rosy glow. I can report that the times I used the products given to me by Dominique Rist, which are divine, they did produce a derriere and thighs that were shiny and pink for several minutes after I rubbed vigorously in pinch-y circular movements as she instructed. No one was privy to my hard work.

I queried every Frenchwoman I know well and even those I casually met in social situations to see if they were vigorously massaging their thighs twice a day, every day. Not one was. A few said they did a little once-a-day rubbing before swimsuit season, but definitely did not continue after August, and they added they had no idea whether it worked physically, although they felt it had psychological benefits.

It was a revelation then to learn that Dr. Fourcade says she actually *does* apply cellulite cream to her thighs, derriere, and stomach *twice* a day and has been doing so for years. "I don't know whether it makes any difference in millimeters; I don't think so," she admitted, "but I know the massage helps circulation and drainage and that's a good thing." I've seen her thighs and she does not have a smidgen of cellulite. She's in her early fifties. We had dinner the other night, and she was wearing a frock several inches above the knee and looked gorgeous. Well, she is gorgeous and is living proof that, basically, there are no (okay, almost no) rules for women of a certain age. Her legs were tan from her summer vacation, which is another anti-cellulite trick.

I was told that cellulite cream works on the occasional pouches under the eyes. I'm testing it. It does seem to work, and Dr. Gallais says there are two ingredients in the products, caffeine and Dextran, a "dermo-cosmetic," that theoretically should help. The sole problem is reactions to fragrances and similar ingredients by the body's most delicate skin. Dextran is a derivative of an exotic bean plant.

Try with caution, or maybe not at all. I had no reaction, but it's not something I really recommend and I don't intend to continue. I prefer my frozen *eau de bleuet*.

HANDS TELL YOU A LOT ABOUT A WOMAN

I had a friend in New York who had beautiful hands. Every Saturday morning, she had a manicure in one of the hundreds of ten-dollar-a-shot pedicure/manicure emporiums. She always wore attention-drawing nail polish. By Wednesday or Thursday, her polish was chipped. Did she simply take a cotton swab and remover to clean up the mess? No, she did not. She didn't seem to care, and yet she had great style in general.

POINT BEING: a natural attribute is instantly destroyed by careless grooming. The rule applies head to toe.

It takes minimal effort to keep hands well-groomed and pretty. Wearing the latest fashion colors takes more time and attention. If the latest hues make you happy, by all means indulge, but at the first sign of a chip, off it comes if repairs are not possible.

Never have I seen chipped polish on either the hands or the feet of a Frenchwoman.

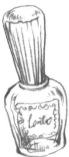

For a softer look—pristine nails with natural white tips (as opposed to a "French manicure," which is not French by the way; it was invented by an American man)—soak fingertips in a cup of warm water with the juice of one lemon and four tablespoons of hydrogen peroxide. An orange stick wrapped in cotton, dipped in the liquid, and swiped under the nails is the perfect finish. At the same time, push down the now-soft cuticles. The addition of the lemon juice, a trick from Elodie, was news to me. Next, a white nail pencil swiped under the tips, and *voilà*. A quick, light—never vigorous—buff or a pale, pale pink polish and you have the low maintenance manicure of the vast majority of Frenchwomen of a certain age.

One of the most valuable lessons I have learned from my French friends and professionals is that many beauty products specifically made for a single purpose can have multiple uses. Take our facial *gommage*, for example; it works wonders on our hands, sloughing and plumping the skin. After the exfoliation, the moisturizing mask provides deep hydration. Hands instantly appear younger.

Let's assume you're rigorous about the care and grooming of your hands. Have you forgotten anything? Do you remember conscientiously to apply a serious SPF formula to them every day? You'll pay for the omission years later if you don't, particularly if you spend an inordinate amount of time driving as I do. The sun streams down onto our hands. Gloves in the winter, major SPF in the summer.

Prepare yourself: bleaching creams for those unfortunate age "freckles" do not work. I can confirm from my own experience, reinforced by Dr. Salort and the doctors Sebban, Gallais, Fourcade, and Serre. Oh, yes, I tried. I spent my money so you can save yours.

If you're troubled enough by brown spots—you notice I'm assiduously avoiding the words "age spots"—and feel they're making you look older, two solutions exist: the expensive one, lasers, and the inexpensive one, liquid nitrogen.

My pal Françoise had her hands and face done with liquid nitrogen at the end of March. Dermatologists will only perform the procedure between October and March because the skin is particularly sensitive to the sun after the intervention.

The procedure "burns" away the brown spots. Françoise told me it didn't hurt in the slightest and the results were really impressive. Her dermatologist gave her a prescription for a special sunblock and she wore, as she would, fingerless gloves for three weeks while the little scabs healed. When she removed her gloves for me, I saw her new, baby-perfect skin. Magic. Dr. Gallais, who is on the cutting edge on all the latest procedures, starts with the liquid nitrogen and if it doesn't work sends her patients to an associate who is an expert with lasers. She says that more than 90 percent of the time the dry ice does the trick and it costs a fraction of the price of the laser.

The liquid nitrogen procedure, better known as cryotherapy or cryosurgery, is, according to my friends, "mildly disagreeable." I did it and found it to be precisely that, mildly disagreeable.

Oh, yes, a local anesthesia is applied before the fun begins.

Fresh, new spots return in place of the old if we're not diligent on the SPF front. Aging is a work in progress after all.

Dr. Sebban offered me a laser treatment. The laser generates an intense beam of light that transfers the energy to a specific spot through a penlike contraption attached to the laser. The light is absorbed by oxyhemoglobin—the red cells carrying oxygen—causing the spots to be destroyed by the heat and leaving healthy cells intact.

An anesthetic cream was applied to my hands prior to the process by her technician. I was in a cushy, comfortable, reclining chair and given goggles to protect my eyes. Up to that moment, all was well with the world. I was told it might be "slightly uncomfortable," but not at all painful. As with everything in life, pain thresholds vary widely, or should I say wildly? The sensation was one of being snapped repeatedly with a big, fat rubber band. The procedure took about thirty minutes, but it seemed like thirty years. The final results—which were excellent, I have to admit—were visible after about two weeks, after the scabs healed.

NEAT FEET

In the United States the typical pedicure is a little foot rub and a slap of polish, but the French believe in a procedure called medical pedicures. These are considered an essential element in a Frenchwoman of a certain age's maintenance regime. For years, they've been part of mine.

After the procedure with sharp, shiny instruments in the hands of a state-licensed professional, my neglected feet are so impeccably beautiful, I can't stop looking at them. Alexandre Lagrande, who has been saving my feet for several years, cuts my toenails to my shape and length specifications; gently scrapes away dead skin, calluses, and budding nasty corns (with above-mentioned sharp, sterile instruments); cleans around each nail; pushes down the cuticles; takes a tiny spinning emery disk to each nail surface, leaving them shiny and smooth; and, for the *grande finale,* gives me a moan-eliciting foot massage with a super-rich foot cream made for that purpose. I make it a point to tell him how much I appreciate the final touch. Usually, he'll throw in a couple more minutes. He makes it a point to tell me to put cream on my feet every night. I always promise I will and sometimes I do.

In France a medical pedicure is less expensive than a *beauté des pieds* (a classic pedicure with polish) and far more satisfying. With continued home maintenance—more on that to come—you can make the investment last for months. If one is diligent, four per year are plenty. If you are planning a visit to France, I recommend you make an appointment. In general they cost between twenty-five and thirty euros.

Truthfully, I can be lazy on the foot front. Estheticians tell me I'm not the only one. Pascale has what I've found to be a pleasant home remedy to get back on our feet. It starts with a footbath of very warm water, a handful of sea salt, and an effervescent aspirin. The aspirin contains salicylic acid, a chemical exfoliant (beta hydroxy acid), and the fizzy part makes it feel festive.

Soak, read, think, relax. Remove feet from the soak, take your body *gommage,* and go to work on the now-soft dead skin; if you feel comfortable with a fine pumice, it's next on the agenda for stubborn calluses. Finally, apply masses of shea or argan butter, cover with clean, white socks, and go to bed.

YOU'RE THINKING: sounds like another chore. Am I right? Don't worry, the remedies work quickly, and you'll be so pleased with your diligence that you'll forget the few minutes it took to get your feet back into "caressable" shape again.

None of the above precludes a *beauté de pieds* with some smashing polish. I wouldn't want you to think my toenails are not polished. Polish on my toes is another one of those details that delights me every day, twelve months a year. Nothing quite like popping out of bed and seeing my happy feet. Some Frenchwomen eschew polish on their feet altogether in the winter, satisfied with their neat feet from their med-ped appointments.

If you're thinking you do not have the time to indulge in the care and maintenance of your skin the way Frenchwomen do, ask yourself these questions: Do I want beautiful skin from head to toe? Do I aspire to look beautiful, perhaps even younger, for my age? Do I feel better about myself when I'm polished and groomed?

Well, of course you do. Who wouldn't? When we feel good about ourselves, we feel powerful, which in turn gives us confidence and, honestly, what is more alluring than a gorgeous façade bolstered by self-assurance? So, please, let me assure you that the time is there if you wish to find it. A few minutes here, a few minutes there—in a month you will have built a series of pleasurable habits. Frenchwomen are every bit as busy as we are, but like everything in life, a woman must choose her priorities.

3

Le Maquillage

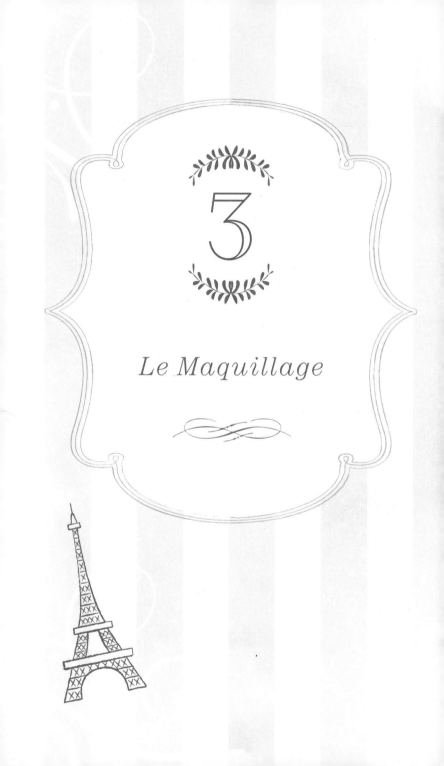

MORE THAN EVER, LESS IS MORE

Never have I met a Frenchwoman who aspires to be someone other than herself. One may admit she wishes she were taller, or that she should have been more conscientious about basking in the sun, but that's it. Frenchwomen, in my experience, do not see any point in trying to change who they are. They prefer the idea of looking the best they can at every age—end of story.

This chapter gave me a dream opportunity. Internationally renowned French makeup artists spent hours explaining to me how cosmetics should be applied for a naturally beautiful effect. They also told me, specifically, which products and colors I should be using. My interviews reinforced my belief that expert advice is a onetime investment that yields immeasurable returns. We should not be using the same cosmetics—and perhaps not the same colors—that we have been using all of our lives. Our skin changes, and most of us change our treatment products as a consequence. It makes sense, then, to re-assess our cosmetics. There are tricks and products on the market specifically designed to enhance the features of women of a certain age, such as foundations with built-in light-reflecting properties.

NATURAL ARTIFICE

Naturel is the mantra of Frenchwomen. They want their hair, their skin, their makeup, their figures, their style, their comportment, and their confidence to appear ever and always *naturel*—an extension of who they are. They also wish us to believe the means to those ends are effortless, but that's another *histoire*.

Olivier Echaudemaison, creative director for Guerlain, echoed a French maxim, saying, "A Frenchwoman understands that each woman is unique. She knows it; she loves it. She has no desire to resemble anyone other than herself. She does not have beauty idols she wishes to emulate. Furthermore, she always wants to seduce, and she knows men are suspicious of obvious artifice."

Artifice is an interesting concept. The word and its meaning are identical in French and English: a clever trick or stratagem; ingenuity; inventiveness; sleight of hand; artless beauty. One understandably might assume that sleight of hand and artless beauty imply subtlety, as in barely there *maquillage*, a little help to enhance one's natural resources perhaps, nothing more.

Certainly that is how the concept is defined today, particularly in regard to Frenchwomen of a certain age, whose makeup appears almost invisible. But that was not always the case in France, where at one time theatrical cosmetic use designated the wearer's station in life and placement inside or outside the court.

During the eighteenth-century reign of Louis XV, cheeks were highly rouged. Courtesans wore a deep, vibrant look-at-me red, while members of the bourgeoisie opted for a clear crimson. Women even wore rouge to bed. Alabaster skin was the norm, and until the beginning of the nineteensth century, the products used to affect the ideal complexion were highly toxic, as their ingredients often included lead, mercury, and arsenic.

At the court of Versailles in the eighteenth century, noblewomen displayed a skin tone that can only be described as *livid*, with rosy cheeks and vermillion lips. As punctuation, they added beauty marks (known as *les mouches*, literally "flies"), cut out of taffeta in whimsical shapes such as stars or half-moons. Often the position of such a beauty mark on a woman's face was a message—the corner of the eye, for example, said "flirtatious" (or even in the mood). *Les mouches* were also employed to cover blemishes.

Amusing in retrospect, despite the perils sometimes involved, and certainly fascinating. Since the dawn of time or, as the French say, "as long as the world has been the world," women have been finding ways to enhance their assets, from grinding up bugs for rouge to juicing berries for scarlet cheeks and lips. I also read long ago that razors were used to "peel"—you see there's nothing new under the sun, only the means to the end—facial skin to reveal the younger and fresher skin below, a surface that could better take on all those dangerous powders. Even today's chemical peels, then, are nothing new—they simply rely on a different means to reach the same end.

Épilation, hair removal, was also an integral part of a lady's *toilette*. To achieve smooth, hairless skin, women used bat or frog's blood, or ants' eggs. I've tried to uncover exactly how these rudimentary "products" were applied—and how successful they were—but to no avail. I simply assume they worked, otherwise it's impossible to imagine doing something so distasteful if it produced no results.

What is most interesting about the past and the present is that during the reign of the kings, women wished to look like one another, copying everything from the color of their lips and the height of their monumental hair constructions to their dresses and accessories.

Today, such a notion is anathema to a Frenchwoman, and it is largely through her radiantly natural embellishment that she underscores her individuality.

That is precisely the effect every Frenchwoman of a certain age hopes to achieve with her skillfully applied *maquillage*. Her artistry is so clever, so flawless that one sees only a lovely, unique, seemingly artifice-free face. Or, as Eric Antoniotti, international artistic and training director for Clarins, put it, "*Vous encore plus belle,*" meaning "you, even more beautiful."

"Every woman has her own personality. Why, then, would she want to look like someone else?" Antoniotti mused. "Frenchwomen are the original versions of themselves."

There you have it, another reason I admire Frenchwomen. They are who they are and that's the way they like it. They decide what will make them look and feel better about *themselves*. It's a simple formula. Many love their cosmetic and treatment products, but they were probably not swayed to buy them because of images the brands used to sell them. Instead, they rely on their dermatologists and sometimes their pharmacists for counsel. Informed advice makes sense to them. Friends gleefully share success stories. What woman doesn't appreciate pretested products endorsed by her girlfriends?

AN IMPECCABLE CANVAS

Clearly, apart from the very basic French aesthetic of enhancing nature with subtle beauty techniques, all would be in vain if the canvas were not impeccable.

A famous French makeup artist, who has traveled the world teaching women how to apply makeup, as well as doing makeup for celebrities and socialites, told me, "I was shocked to meet mothers outside of France who were encouraging their daughters to use cover-up products instead of making appointments with dermatologists to solve simple skin problems. It seems to me that contacting a doctor would help a girl build a lifetime of confidence and develop good habits. It's so negative to cover up, as if there is something wrong with her. It's encouraging her to hide the problem rather than requesting a straightforward treatment from a doctor," he said.

It's true. French girls learn from an early age, under the tutelage of *mère* and *grand-mère*, that flawless skin is among the world's most enduring beauty secrets.

Mère and *grand-mère* probably also warn the little ones about the dangers of too much sun exposure without proper protection and the destructive results of cigarette smoking and excessive alcohol intake. Clearly, many have blithely ignored this advice, Brigitte Bardot among them. But we are not here to discuss the unfortunate recklessness of youth. No, our *raison d'être* is to examine closely the good habits that pay off for the duration.

One of my friends, who still smokes and spent her youth baking in the blistering rays of Saint-Tropez—and has the skin to show for it—uses herself as an example to her daughter of what *not* to do if she doesn't wish to look significantly older than her years. As a result, Caroline applies sunscreen liberally and doesn't smoke. She has tried unsuccessfully on numerous occasions to convince her mother to quit.

When women have taken meticulous care of their skin, it shows; it glows. If the skin beneath the makeup is not flawless, what's the point of applying layers of product and patchwork cover-ups?

No Frenchwoman of a certain age says to herself, "*Eh, oui*, I certainly hope my friends, family, and everyone I meet will love the way I applied my makeup today."

Indeed, I sincerely doubt that is any woman's objective, no matter what her nationality. "Sleight of hand" implies "light of hand," as in "imperceptible," as in *totalement naturel*. Who would ever seek compliments for well-applied cosmetics? At best, we might be pleased a friend notices our new lipstick color.

Too much makeup, particularly foundation and camouflage products, is not only unnatural, off-putting, and old-fashioned, but it also makes a face of a certain age look older. Heavy makeup sinks into wrinkles and pores. When Frenchwomen of a certain age apply foundation, we do not see it.

Frenchwomen know that modern makeup is not created to hide lines; its function is to help us look fresh and glow with the appearance of good health. My friends and acquaintances, including my doctors, never obsess over wrinkles. "It's not natural *not* to have them," one doctor friend told me. "In fact, it's terrifying to see women who try to hide lines and wrinkles with either surgery or cosmetics. Honestly, I have no problem with mine."

She's in her early fifties and stunning and she does have lines on her lovely, usually lightly tanned, face. I've known her since she was in her twenties, and I find her prettier today than ever.

Frenchwomen understand intrinsically that one does not trifle with one's natural resources. Our faces are our fortune, so to speak, which is why Frenchwomen devote time and attention to daily rituals that keep their skin immaculate and radiant.

LE MAQUILLAGE

Frenchwomen prize a fresh, unaffected appearance that adds to their age-defying allure. Therefore, nowhere do they apply more subtle artistry than with their *maquillage*. As young girls, they may have played with crazily colorful eye shadows, glitter, and blue lipstick, but that was just for fun. As women, they want to underscore subtly and enhance their features so their best selves shine through.

"Let's be clear," Olivier Echaudemaison said, "all Frenchwomen above a certain age use foundation. I associate foundation with lingerie. Both reassure and give a woman confidence, both are worn first and foremost for her; they are her little secrets."

Adopting a French mindset when performing a daily grooming routine that might otherwise seem mundane truly does change one's outlook on life. I've always enjoyed the process of putting on makeup, particularly for a party, but putting on my underwear was simply what I did before I put on my clothes. Now I like thinking of both of these gestures as exquisitely feminine, personal, and morale boosting. Mind over matter can be a remarkable confidence builder.

Maybe it's psychological, maybe it's silly, but I can't help being drawn to these French notions of putting a positive, feminine, take-pleasure-in-the-moment spin on the quotidian. That's what I was thinking as Eric Antoniotti was showing me how to choose and apply foundation. I'll get to that in a moment.

You may think a no-makeup look suggests, literally, not wearing makeup, but nothing could be further from reality.

"Too much is the greatest makeup misstep any woman can employ to look older and no makeup does more or less the same thing—no color, no light, no enhancement." *Et voila*, there we have Olivier Echaudemaison's take on the subject.

"For Frenchwomen, it's all about nuances," Echaudemaison continued. "And to admit to taking time to apply makeup is unthinkable. A compliment about how wonderful a friend looks might, at most, elicit a swift response of 'Oh, it's just a touch of Terracotta, *chérie.*'" (Terracotta is the iconic compact bronzing powder from Guerlain that comes in scores of tones for every skin color and really does make one look rested with a just-back-from-vacation glow.)

"A Frenchwoman can be sipping a glass of wine while she tells you she's not drinking," Echaudemaison said, laughing, "and you believe her!"

Let me break down my lessons for you.

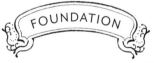

FOUNDATION

The first question every woman asks is "How do I choose the right color?"

Never mind trying to use the famous wrist test. "The blue of the veins makes it impossible," Olivier Echaudemaison said.

How about this trick from Eric Antoniotti: the palms of our hands. Really? You need a friend or two for the test. I did it with two women during our interview. We all thought it was great fun, though bizarre. He told us to turn our hands over, palms up. Two of us had very rosy skin, and the other had a sort of peachy cast to her skin. The result: the woman and I with the rose-colored palms need a yellow-based foundation, while the woman with the more orange tone should look for a rose-based foundation. "Opposites balance and color-correct," Antoniotti said.

Yellow is for éclat and rose is for freshness; both are necessary, Antoniotti added.

Texture tends to be a personal choice; I like liquids.

I have the impression that no makeup artist really expects, although they may hope, women will apply their base with a brush or one of those purpose-made sponges the professionals use. Thinking this attitude might be another example of my American *laisser-aller*, I asked a couple of my French girlfriends how they applied their makeup. "With my fingers," they all replied.

I've started applying my foundation with a brush when I'm feeling ambitious. It's worth learning the technique (not complicated, but not habit either). The result is barely there because of feathery strokes and, to my surprise, the product goes on quickly and evenly.

I've always used foundation, but never all over my face, only on my nose, a dot on my forehead, around my eyes, and a dab on my chin. According to the experts, that's all you need. Don't you just love positive reinforcement? After they helped me solve the color conundrum, I admitted that I often wondered whether my application technique needed improvement.

This is how it's done they told me: dab, dab, dab where you think you want foundation (no, it's not necessary all over the face; who does that anyway?), gently blend, no boundary lines. Here comes the secret: place your warm hands on your face and lightly press where makeup has been applied. It is now perfectly "set"— and immaculately *naturel*.

My dermatologist, Valerie Gallais, mixes day moisturizing cream with a squirt of self-tanning product in the palm of her hand, and that is her foundation. "Then I add a touch of powder," she said. I can attest to the fact it doesn't look like she has anything to camouflage. If she does, mission accomplished.

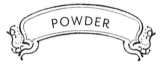

POWDER

I don't know about you, but I've always been afraid of powder, and until recently, as in the last year, I had never used it. Powdered blush, yes; powdered eye shadow, yes; powdered bronzer, sometimes; powdered eyebrow enhancer, not so much, as I prefer a pencil. But I had never used translucent powder, even though it sounded tantalizingly seductive. I avoided the temptation. Most Frenchwomen of a certain age use powder, albeit sparingly. It's the sophisticated finish to natural makeup.

Finally, thanks to Eric Antoniotti, I now know how to use translucent powder. He pointed out the important distinction between shine and glow. (I knew the difference, actually, but didn't know what to do about it, which is the crux of the matter.) When an invisible veil of powder is properly applied, the skin beneath it glows, he promised.

Then, he took a medium-sized brush, stroked it across a powder compact, shook off most of the contents, and gently swept the brush over my forehead and down my nose and then flicked the merest whisper on my chin. Result: a no-powder look, exactly what I assume every article I've ever read on the subject was trying to explain, and what every woman who uses powder learned years ago.

Like just about every Frenchwoman I know, I, too, am hooked on those divine bronzing powders that make us look healthy and sun-kissed, particularly if they have a smattering of illuminating whatsits in them. Olivier Echaudemaison chose the right color for me—there is one out there for every skin tone, from dark to light—took a huge brush and gently whisked it across my forehead, over my nose, onto my cheekbones, onto the tip of my chin and under my jawline. I assumed he was giving me a *trompe-l'oeil* neck lift with the last swipe. I hoped it would work.

When choosing the color from the zillions—I never exaggerate—of gradations of tone and illumination, I suggest a conference with an expert. Bronzer is not a product to buy on instinct. I tried on my own a couple of years ago, and I managed to create an effect I imagine no one wants—a dirty face. The powder was strategically placed and artfully applied, but the effect was ridiculous, not to mention expensive.

Now that we've established the foundation/powder rituals and confirmed that they exist, the next steps in front of the mirror are the personal details, like the accessories in a wardrobe that make a look unique: mascara, eyeliner, lipstick and, most likely, a hint of blush.

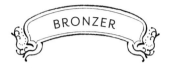

BRONZER

A sun-kissed look—accomplished either cosmetically or intelligently with sun exposure using proper SPF products—is one many Frenchwomen covet. It says vacation, tropical islands, ski slopes, Saint-Tropez, Brittany.

In the past, though, having the slightest tan was out of the question for women of a certain stature. Tanned skin implied a woman was a peasant; a ghostly white face announced she was a lady of leisure. During the time of the Sun King, Louis XIV, when women of the court were obliged to participate in promenades, they wore masks over their faces to protect them from exposure to the sun. These masks were held in place by clenching a button between one's teeth. (There were actually two advantages to this bizarre custom: masks ensured that skin remained porcelain-like, and the ladies were exempt from participating in the exhausting exercise of clever repartee.)

It wasn't until the start of the twentieth century that a tan began to indicate something quite different: a sunny holiday, good health, natural beauty.

I finally know how to apply *bronzé* powders, and even an alternative darker foundation to give me the look of a light tan, which I never would have had the courage to try before Olivier Echaudemaison chose the color and showed me how to use it, just like a Frenchwoman does.

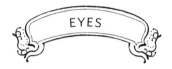

EYES

Catherine de Médicis, the formidable Italian wife of Henri II, is credited with introducing mascara, defined brows, and a blurred eyeliner/shadow effect to the French court. For those of us in the twenty-first century, the rule is one coat of mascara for day, two for evening, lashes brushed before and after application.

Clumpy eyelashes announce two possibilities: you're wearing mascara and those lovely lashes are not natural or, worse, you can't see well enough without your glasses to unclump them.

Subtle eyeliner—a fine line close to the upper lashes (most agree not on the lower rims), with the outer end of the line turned up slightly in a comma turned on its side. The comma should be applied *before* the eye is lined so it does not become a thick extension, but rather a light lift. I just learned this trick, and I only use the comma for the evening. It definitely lifts the eye, if subtly.

The majority of my friends line their eyes. I did for years, stopped for at least a decade, and have now restarted.

Eyebrows are well tended because, as every woman knows, they frame the face, and when a dab of highlighter is applied under the arch, the eye is instantly lifted. Olivier told me that with age our eyes grow—I'm not sure that's the appropriate word—closer together, and, therefore, we must put a dot of highlighter on each of the inner corners to make them appear wider apart. He said that if we look at a picture of ourselves at twelve years old and another today, we would see the phenomenon. "That dot re-opens the eyes like magic," he said. Yes, it does.

Another step for most of us: when we look tired and don't have the time for more serious treatment tricks, one of the many liquid wand highlighters included in every makeup collection works wonders when applied beneath the eye from the inside corner and dot, dot, dotting to the outside edge with a pat, pat, pat finish. And don't forget—an eyelash curler is a mini eyelift. I've been using an eyelash curler ever since I first found one on my mother's dressing table next to her Helena Rubinstein red lipstick and her unforgettably beautiful bottle of Arpège perfume when I was about eight.

No matter how many times I beseeched him, Olivier Echaudemaison declined to cover up the dark circles under my eyes, and it wasn't as if he didn't have all the products at his disposal. We were, after all, in the Guerlain headquarters. He insisted they were natural. I knew they were natural, but I wanted to hide them. He said he liked them. I hate them.

In the nineteenth century, women supposedly forced themselves to sleep as little as possible to create dark circles naturally. When that didn't work, they drew lines around their eyes. At least by that time they had stopped powdering their faces with finely ground toxic metals. Instead, they drank liters of vinegar and lemon juice to make their complexions pallid; that was intended to exaggerate the contrast between their dark, sunken, tired eyes and their faces. Emma Bovary, you may recall, drank vinegar to enhance her pallor. Looking ill was in.

One of the first urban legends I heard when we moved to France was that dark circles, even those accompanied by loathsome bags, implied a woman had an interesting life, as in a busy nightlife, if you see what I mean.

I maintain that one can have an interesting nightlife and still look fresh in the morning with a little help from her cosmetic friends.

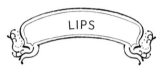

LIPS

Every woman needs two lipsticks, the experts agree. They should be in the rose family—there is a rose, bunches of roses actually, out there for every woman—a lighter shade for day, a deeper, richer tone for evening.

So many perfectly innocent subjects or objects take on sexual connotations in France, which I've come to understand is more of a joke than anything else. Take lipstick, for example.

French magazines explain how to find the perfect rose: they tell us it's the shade we see when our lips have been "lightly bitten." How's that for a sensual reference?

In the eighteenth century, the color of a woman's lips indicated her social position. Among *les dames de la court*, pomegranate was the predominant color; among the bourgeoisie, it was a clear red; violet was reserved for women with dubious reputations. Perhaps the choice of a vibrant violet was a form of advertising; otherwise, it seems strange that a woman would have chosen to announce her questionable virtue.

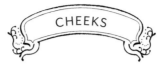

CHEEKS

Even the words have changed over time. Once we said "rouge," today we say "blush" to indicate the slightest hint of color—the natural flush of color that spreads across our cheeks when we blush.

Cream or powder? The experts indicate powder, because they believe it's easier to control and gives a lighter finish. Many women, particularly those who have wrinkled cheeks (I know, I know), prefer cream.

THE EXCEPTIONS, THE INDIVIDUALISTS

Some Frenchwomen have established their indelible signature looks by breaking all the rules. Red, red lips are often involved in the individual looks that underscore a woman's personality. My pal Françoise and the late, famous interior architect Andrée Putman fall into this category. Others use kohl eyeliner to achieve *les oeils de biche* (doe eyes). Those details are extensions of style and personality, and I love that notion.

My friend Françoise would not be Françoise without her bright, matte crimson lips and orangey-red hair, a color that is not part of any palette that ever occurred to Mother Nature. Madame Putman, with her strong features, parchment skin, graphically severe hairstyle, and stark, clean geometric wardrobe punctuated the overall effect with her startling lip color. Chantal Thomass, famous for her lingerie designs, is another red-lipstick fan. Again, it's part of

The Secrets of
LE MAQUILLAGE

Let me share with you, then, what I've learned about *maquillage* while living in France:

1) USE A PRIMER. It takes only seconds and changes everything: I've started using Clarins Baume Beauté Eclair (Beauty Flash Balm), which I apply between my day cream and foundation. It provides "radiance in a flash," just as the tube claims.

2) TRY IT FIRST. Frenchwomen rarely buy any type of cosmetic product without first asking for a sample to take home to try under various lighting conditions, like testing paint on a wall.

3) BRIGHTEN YOUR EYES WITH MAKEUP ARTISTS' SECRET WEAPON: Gouttes Bleues from Innoxa. Deep blue, plant-based eye drops, they make the whites of the eyes brilliantly clear and rested-looking.

4) USE THE SPACE BETWEEN THE TOP OF THE WRIST AND THE BASE OF THE THUMB as a makeup palette. This makes application infinitely easier.

5) DON'T WASTE PRODUCTS. Eric Antoniotti told me to put a half-pump quantity of makeup on my palette (in other words, don't press the pump all the way down), and if more is needed, add a quarter-pump's worth. I've never needed more than a half.

6) USE THE PALMS OF YOUR HANDS to fix makeup as the final step. Press lightly. The effect is your skin, only better. Guaranteed.

7) CHOOSING A FOUNDATION COLOR ONE COLOR LIGHTER than our skin tone tends to make us look younger. A foundation color one shade darker, on the other hand, looks healthy, like we're just back from the slopes. Too dark a tone is aging, so test first. Most Frenchwomen opt to take the powder *bronzé* route; it's much easier and "safer."

8) A CLEVER WAY TO TEST A BASE COLOR is to put it on your nose to judge whether it is too light or too dark for continuity.

9) APPLY LIQUID BASE with a brush for a fast and fastidious finish.

10) "EVERY WOMAN SHOULD HAVE a rose blush compact in her *sac*. It's a sort of security," Antoniotti said. "Rosy blushes make the face look fresh and less tired."

11) DARK LIPSTICK COLORS emphasize wrinkles. Instead, have two lipsticks in the rose range: lighter for day, deeper for night. Logical, *non*?

12) SELECT A LIP LINER the same color as your lipstick or apply your lipstick with a brush made for that purpose. Both guarantee precise application and an immaculate finish.

13) TO ERASE FATIGUE INSTANTLY, Echaudemaison suggests putting highlighter on the corners of the nose and lips. He noted, "Lips tend to turn down over time; light lifts them."

14) A FIVE-MINUTE MAKEUP ROUTINE includes day cream, primer, foundation, curl lashes, correct brows, one coat of mascara, blush if necessary, lip color—go.

15) AND MY VERY FAVORITE LESSON: Never repair your makeup in public. *Jamais, jamais, jamais*—never, never, never. As my friend Anne-Françoise remarked, "Anything that has to do with beauty is done in private."

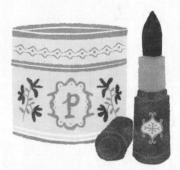

who she is, with her shiny black hair, razor-cut bangs, and mostly black-and-white wardrobe.

For these women, statement lip color serves as a bold accessory that is so much a part of their essence that age is irrelevant. They have created indelible, unforgettable images.

"Americans read and ask questions," one beauty expert told me. "Frenchwomen try for themselves." (She also told me that if a salesperson pays a Frenchwoman a compliment, chances are she won't buy anything. "We hate it when salespeople give us a compliments," she said.)

FRAGRANCE

It would be impossible to speak about the facets of visual beauty, subtle though they may be, without also examining the captivating aura of fragrance. Makeup and fragrance have been inextricably intertwined throughout the ages. They coexist naturally.

When one thinks about French women, two images come instantly to mind: perfume and lingerie. And, as one famous French perfume "nose" (the informal designation for a perfume designer) observed, "When the lights are off and romance is in the air, our senses are heightened and it is skin and perfume that excite us." Perfume, he went on to say, "can make us fall in love."

I think Coco Chanel had a point when she proclaimed, "A woman who doesn't wear perfume has no future."

Catherine de Médicis introduced still more refinement to the French court when a leather tanner in Grasse, Monsieur Galimard, gave her a pair of gloves scented with perfume. Because hides that were tanned to make fine leather products—from shoes to fashionable accessories, notably belts, gloves, and small bags—had an appalling odor, the addition of fragrance was an extraordinarily ingenious development. She began wearing her sweet-smelling gloves, and the court soon followed her lead. She was, in many ways, a daring fashion leader.

As with every aspect of humanity, myths, mysteries and manners dictated the mode of the times. During the eighteenth century, the French court was considered the height of elegance and refinement, and heady fragrances contributed to that reputa-

"Americans read and ask questions, Frenchwomen try for themselves."

tion—whereas hygiene as we know it had no relevance. Prior to the eighteenth century, the only parts of the body that were regularly washed were the hands and the face. The face and hands were cleansed with scented water, while the mouth was rinsed. Foul odors from unwashed bodies were covered with strong perfumes, such as musk, jasmine, amber, tuberose, and various combinations thereof. The nineteenth century heralded an epoch that embraced nature and all that was natural, including water and, consequently, bathing.

No matter what unpleasant circumstances led to the creation of perfume initially, today it exists for the purpose of pure pleasure, which it certainly elicits.

Fragrance is highly individual, yet it is another extension of a woman's personality, and when it mingles with her skin, it becomes her own. Although fragrance existed for centuries, it was the French who refined the fine art of perfumery and are credited with creating the modern-day perfume industry. Therefore, it is not surprising that when we think of a Frenchwoman, we think of perfume.

Fragrance is inescapable and often unforgettable. The faintest trace of perfume can carry us unbidden to long forgotten memories. A never-before-experienced fragrance can draw us in with its redolent promise. It is invisible, and it speaks to us sometimes in ways we do not understand.

Just as makeup is used today by Frenchwomen to look and feel confident—themselves, only better—perfume, too, is an extension of their personalities. I asked Serge Lutens, considered one of the world's most gifted perfume creators ever, why perfume is important for a woman.

He told me, "Perfume reactivates the memory of ourselves. It's clear that a perfume is important [only] when the woman who wears it recognizes herself in it and it becomes part of her."

Lutens perfectly captured a French-woman's view of herself when he famously observed, "Perfume is . . . a choice made in the first person, the dot on the *i*." That says it all, *n'est-ce pas*?

Most of my French friends have worn the same perfumes for decades. For each, the chosen scent has created that indelible connection to memory. A few do dabble in new fragrances, many times received as gifts, but ultimately they tend to return to their signature scents. Often, a perfume marks a moment in a woman's life when she was happiest, perhaps when she met the love of her life. "My husband says he knows me by my perfume," a friend of mine said. When her perfume was discontinued, she was miserable, but finally she found something new. "It's almost as if I'm embarking on another phase of my life," she said. "It's silly, but the transition was traumatic."

Francis Kurkdjian is the "nose" behind a collection of exotic, divine fragrances under his eponymous label, as well as scents for Jean Paul Gaultier, Narciso Rodriguez, Christian Dior with Hedi Slimane, Lanvin, and Elie Saab.

"Perfume is fascinating because it creates emotion," he explained. "It's mysterious because it is invisible and yet inescapable."

As with makeup, the experts advise a woman who has not found and stayed with a signature fragrance throughout her life to request a sample and live with it before she commits. "She may fall in love with the top note in a perfume store, but she must wear it around the clock for a couple of days. It's also important that the people in her life who are most important to her like her perfume. Otherwise, it—and she—will be repellent to them," Kurkdjian said.

Trying before buying, as we saw with *le maquillage*, is a very French approach to all aspects of beauty. Frenchwomen ask for samples of everything from treatment products to perfume. They want to live with and experience a new item before they commit.

"Perfume is a gift we give not only to ourselves, but to others. Sometimes we are unaware of the recipient of this gift," Kurkdjian said.

How true that is. I've often passed a woman who gave me the gift of her perfume on a Paris street. On occasion, I've been tempted to follow one of those women and ask, "What is it that you're wearing?" But I never have. I appreciate the moment and continue on my way.

The French double-cheek air kiss offers a unique opportunity to accept graciously a perfume *cadeau* from either a man or a woman. One of my favorite colognes is My-Reason-For-Living-In-France's signature fragrance, Pour Monsieur by Chanel. Whenever I travel for more than a week, I take tiny spritz samples with me so that I can smell him while we're apart.

My daughter Andrea's grown-up introduction to "real" fragrance was Chanel No. 19. I think she received her first bottle when she was fourteen. Had I met Francis Kurkdjian earlier, she would have had her initial experience at eight.

Kurkdjian had a genius idea while watching his beloved niece Agathe play. He decided to make simple, one-note scents in the form of bubbles. The concept is to initiate little girls into the wonders of fragrance. The collection includes four scents: violet, pear, cut grass, and mint, all appropriately colored to make them even more appealing. Here's what you do: open the bottle, fill the circle in the wand with the liquid (you remember, don't you?), blow *bulles*, and then walk through the bubbles as they burst with fragrance.

Frédéric Malle, the famous "editor of perfumes," as he calls himself, said he has found that women tend to be drawn naturally to fragrances that are enhanced by their complexions. Fragrance is so personal, apparently, that it is basically instinctual.

Fragrance is no doubt associated with romance and seduction because—unlike makeup—it's unseen and the reactions it can evoke are often inexplicable.

Thus the most obvious question: Where and how should a woman apply her perfume?

One woman asked Francis Kurkdjian if he thought she should spray her perfume behind her knees so that the scent would rise. "I forced myself not to say, 'That's ridiculous,'" he recalled.

There seems to be a consensus that perfume sprayed lightly in the hair (granted probably not on the beach in the summer) is a delightful option. Movement and air diffuse perfume.

Never mind the theories, techniques, and debates: a woman should spray or dab perfume "wherever she wants to be kissed," as Coco Chanel famously declared.

All the men I consulted agreed.

There is no better way to conclude this chapter than by telling you what Eric Antoniotti said to me right before we performed a double-cheek kiss and exchanged our *au revoirs*: "It's a privilege to be a woman; every woman should abuse that privilege. Forget the past. Do everything according to love, pleasure, and passion."

Seriously, you've got to *adore* the French. Encouraging the pursuit of love, pleasure, and passion as a philosophy for life is the best beauty advice we could possibly receive. Just add perfume, pink blush, and attitude.

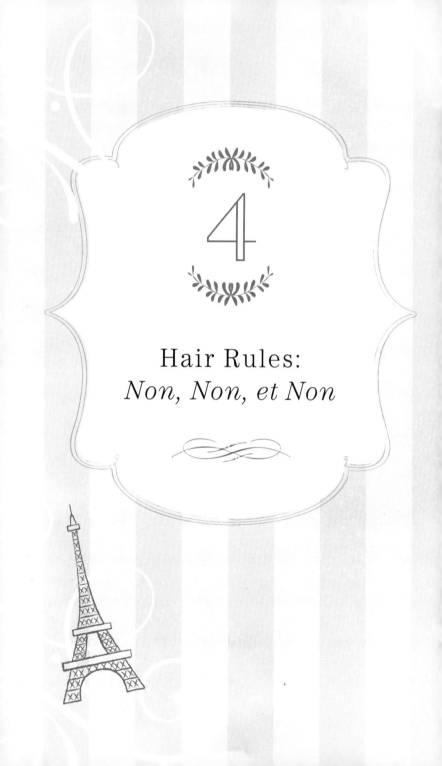

4

Hair Rules:
Non, Non, et Non

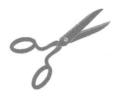

CUT, COLOR, CARE (AND A FEW SURPRISES)

Arguably, one of a Frenchwoman's most remarkable natural resources is her thick, bouncy, healthy hair.

Apart from her enviable figure, which may or may not come naturally, I think her hair is largely responsible for her international reputation as a creature of unparalleled elegance.

Why do I think this? Primarily because her hair *moves*. In the world over, young women have shiny, swingy hair, but after a certain age, many women want their tresses to stay in place. Neat and practical inexorably replace natural. What a shame.

French women of a certain age reign supreme in this extremely important grooming detail. Their hair is never fussy or fixed; a breeze may lift it carelessly and they don't care. It's another attractive aspect of their seeming nonchalance. Their coiffures add to an attitude that makes them appear young and carefree.

Why is this possible? Because a Frenchwoman has taken the time and effort and passed through the necessary trial-and-error tribulations to find the one person who can give her the absolutely perfect haircut and color, which she knows will make her look and feel confident and comfortable every day, no matter what. Frenchwomen know what they want, but as for all of us, it sometimes takes considerable time and dedication to find stylists who can execute their desires.

As I've said, we are our own best investment. We must never forget this truism. Once we accept this very French idea, we acknowledge that investments require attention and active intervention. Sometimes, you need to invest more than time. You may need to invest money. So, let me be perfectly clear: Your hair *is* you. You wake up in the morning, you look in the mirror, and you see that wonderful cut and color. Instantly, you feel good about yourself before you start your day. That's a major payoff from an investment, and no one knows this better than Frenchwomen of a certain age. Budgeting for one's well-being and self-confidence is serious business. There are many areas in which one can be aggressively frugal, and others—haircuts and color, for example—in which one should accept that she must make a relatively important budget outlay. No matter their means, Frenchwomen do not like to squander their time or money, but when it comes to their hair, they tend to be extravagant.

A Frenchwoman also does not face the dreaded daily hair ritual of shampoo, conditioner, product, the blow-dry contortion of torturing her hair into a "do" that the cut and natural inclination of the hair may resist, followed by more product to hold it in position. Under normal conditions, Frenchwomen wash their hair twice a week. That's a beauty secret if there ever was one. My hair looks best two days after a shampoo; that's when it cooperates with whatever I want it to do. I admit, I'm not very demanding, since all I do is brush my hair. After a swim, I rinse it and add a leave-in conditioner, avoiding the scalp area and concentrating on the ends.

As one of my French friends pointed out, "We don't want 'sophisticated,' because anything 'too-too' seems contrived, and we *always* want everyone to think that everything we do is effortless, completely natural."

That's another one of their secrets: Frenchwomen of a certain age will blatantly deny that they've spent time fixing themselves up, and the best part is that they all know it's not quite true. It's an inside joke.

Some Frenchwomen have weekly brushings built into their beauty budgets. "After having my hair done—by that I mean a wash and a blow-dry—I feel so confident and groomed that I think it's worth the expense," one of my particularly chic friends told me. She deep-conditions her hair at home, but for her, these weekly indulgences are worth every *centime*.

TO CUT OR NOT TO CUT:
THAT IS NO LONGER THE QUESTION

The predominant question *inside* every woman's head is this: how long is too long after age fifty? It's a dilemma for all of us. While the pros say length and birthdays are not inextricably bound, I see few Frenchwomen of a certain age with hair below their shoulders. Almost no French actresses, television journalists, friends, or women on the street have opted for the current American approach to super-long hair after a certain age. However, shoulder-length locks are often the norm. As my hairstylist, Michelle, said, "My clients rarely want that 'break' at the shoulders; they prefer their hair mid-length or at that stage where there is just a bit of air—read: light—between shoulders and coif."

For years, I've been taking pictures of women of a certain age in Paris and near my home in the countryside for my blog. Some in their forties have styles below their shoulders, but definitely not *long*. The vast majority have various degrees of mid-length bobs. And think about French actresses for a moment: not one has hair trailing down her back, or flipped over her shoulders in front.

Valérie Trierweiler, France's "First Companion" (the partner of France's president, François Hollande) is the single most visible exception to the supposed "rule" against extremely long hair after forty-five. Former model and ex-First Lady Carla Bruni-Sarkozy has also had long hair in her forties.

If you look at pictures of Catherine Deneuve when she was in her twenties and thirties, you'll see that her thick, ultra-blonde mane was often below her shoulders, and it was sublime. Today it seems obvious how aging that length would be on her. At one point she tried a short bob, which had the fashion press abuzz with the news, but she quickly let it grow back to a classic, versatile not-quite-shoulder-length style. Still, then and now, she can wear her hair up in a soft do and it is eternally flattering.

Many years ago, singer and actress Françoise Hardy cut her girlishly long, straight hair into a sexy short bob with lush bangs that fell alluringly into her eyes—and at the same time she decided to go gray. She looks amazing. Jeanne Moreau cut her hair with layers for softness. And what about Jane Birkin, beloved and emulated as a style icon in her adopted France? She went from her signature long, long, mod rod-straight hair to the sweet pixie cut she sports today.

As near as I can tell by perusing decades of photographs, Inès de la Fressange, Anouk Aimée, and Fanny Ardant have almost exactly the same hairstyles they've had forever, give or take a slight tweak here and there. All chose lengths that were, and remain, above their shoulders.

Still, Parisian hairstylists maintain that there are no rules for length and age. Basically, I agree with their pronouncement in principle.

Age may or may not play into the decision to take scissors to our hair after a major birthday. Long, short, or in-between, a hairstyle is perhaps the single most important extension of a woman's outward personality. Will she look better, more soignée, younger if she cuts? Maybe. Maybe not. None of the hairstylists I interviewed felt long was wrong if it was right for the individual.

In one of my many file folders, I discovered a *New York Times* article from 2005 heralding the freedom and femininity that women in their late forties, fifties, and beyond attributed to their long locks. Sexuality plays into the decision as well, the article went on to say. Hair is a "sexy accessory," as one fashion editor put it. On the practical side, it was noted that extra-long hair can have dual yet opposite benefits: it provides a protective veil to conceal wrinkles and creases, or to hide plastic surgery scars. Talk about a win-win.

Again, to cut or not to cut is an individual decision and yet another means for a woman to express her personality.

THERE ARE NO RULES

"It's impossible to have rules about a woman and her hair," Bernard Friboulet, owner of the couldn't-be-more-divinely-insider-feeling salon Très Confidentiel, said. "What is more personal, more all about a woman than her hair?"

Friboulet recently cut Chanel's external relations director Marie-Louise de Clermont-Tonnerre's hair into a wispy, saucy bob. Always stunning, she looks prettier than ever. Before he took her shorter, for as long as I've known her, which is at least twenty-five years, her hair had been elegantly cut into a versatile mid-length style.

"I take my time working with my clients, particularly when they think they want to make drastic changes," Friboulet told me as he dashed back and forth between our interview and a woman in mid-decision. "Often there are myriad reasons why women want to 'change their heads,' and they don't necessarily have anything to do with style or fashion. Sometimes it's more complicated, an emotional decision, and I understand that. That's why I like to spend time with them," he explained.

For as long as I've known my friend Anne-Françoise, she has had an easy-care pixie cap of super-short, shiny blonde layers. She has often played with the color, experimenting with scores of nuances of blonde and, to my great surprise, she was a redhead for our wedding. She looked great in all her hues. She chose the style because it was easy and feminine.

A few years ago, she made a different styling decision. She let her pixie spikes grow longer. It was a brilliant move on her part. She still has a wash-and-go cut, but the overall effect is softer, kinder, much more flattering.

The famous celebrity coiffeur Alexandre Zouari keeps Marisa Berenson's long, luxurious, wildly curly tresses glossy and free-flowing. He agrees with Friboulet.

"It's finished; there are no rules," he proclaimed. "I think it might be interesting if a woman wants to try something new, but an obligatory cut at a certain age, sometimes yes, but often *non, non, non*. Marisa Berenson has made the right decision for her hair. The style *is* Marisa Berenson."

I couldn't agree with him more. One day while having tea with Berenson, one of the greatest models of all time, I realized that it would be impossible to imagine her without her lush, gorgeous tresses. They're part of her personality, her style, her stunningly original nonconformist approach to fashion that seems to be in her genes. Actually, it probably *is* in her genes, since her grandmother was the eccentric, avant-garde, creative designer Elsa Schiaparelli.

Some stylists did equivocate about the to cut or not to

cut dilemma. Many mentioned that hair that falls below the shoulder or that breaks at the shoulder is not the best decision for many women. It works for Berenson because her hair seems airy and almost careless, and she often sweeps it back at the sides, up, and away from her lovely face.

The most important lesson of all when it comes to the to-cut-or-not-to-cut decision? It's simple, the experts agree: whatever makes a woman feel good about herself.

THE COLOR CONUNDRUM

I have a friend who colors her chin-length blunt-cut hair herself. Her coif has no nuances of tone. It's dark brown, almost black—always has been and, I assume, always will be. When she has white roots peeking through, she takes out a toothbrush and has her husband touch up the offenders with her allover color. She claims she does take deep conditioning seriously. I believe her.

She is the only friend I know who is into do-it-yourself hair color. Meanwhile, my highlights are a complicated affair. It took me literally years to finally find a colorist who would listen to me. I found her after I met a woman at a cocktail party who had exactly the tone-on-tone-on-tone blondeness I was seeking. She sent me directly to Michelle.

My advice, and that of my French girlfriends, is to find the best coiffeur you can afford and accept the fact that trial and error in this domain will be worth the pain. Go ahead, stop a woman on the street who has the color and/or the cut of your dreams. I once worked up my nerve and did just that in Paris, and the woman couldn't have been kinder. She actually took out a piece of paper and wrote down the name and address of her coiffeur. Wouldn't you be flattered if someone asked you?

Once you've budgeted for cut and color, you can do the rest yourself—rinses, conditioners, masques, deep-heat treatments, etc. Masques and deep-heat treatments, vigorously recommended by the experts, are part of my regular home routine, and the results are worth the effort, particularly with all the above-mentioned highlighting that I can't live without. If I didn't sleep with deep, deep, through-the-night conditioner applied, I'm sure my hair wouldn't have the glistening shine it does.

Now, let's talk more about color, which I did with two of the world's most famous colorists: Christophe Robin and Rodolphe. The latter probably has a last name, but he did not divulge it in our interview.

The international fashion press considers them to be artists, and based on their roster of famous clients and the women I've seen sitting in their salons, that seems a fair assessment of their talents. They do listen; obviously with their experience and their creative approach to color, they help women find the shades that will flatter their eyes and skin color.

Christophe Robin did not really approve of my *balayage,* while Rodolphe said it was "*pas mal*" (not bad). Both offered to fix me up. To date I haven't taken them up on their offers, though I am tempted.

Priceless Lessons
FROM THE EXPERTS

This is what I learned from Christophe Robin, who counts Catherine Deneuve, Isabelle Adjani, Tilda Swinton, Faye Dunaway, Beyoncé, Claudia Schiffer, Emmanuelle Béart, Kristin Scott Thomas, and Juliette Binoche among his clients:

✧ The day before coloring your hair, apply a deep-moisturizing masque, and do not wash it out before heading to your colorist.

✧ For women over forty, no matter what color their hair, golden tones—appropriate for the base color—add warmth, which by extension makes their faces appear younger.

✧ Eyebrows are normally the color that most closely match one's natural hair color.

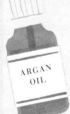

✧ When choosing color, it's best to go no more than one or two shades lighter or darker. "It's true that 80 percent of women ask to go lighter than their natural color, even when they shouldn't," he added. (Yes, I'm admitting my transgression.)

✧ After five consecutive shampoos, one should deep-condition colored hair. Put on a plastic shower cap, and over that wrap a heated towel to amp up the efficacy of the treatment. (The plastic shower cap not only seals in the heat, but also keeps the product on the hair and not absorbed into the towel. I never thought of that.)

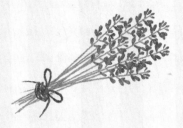

→ Many women believe—falsely—that if they go much lighter, they will look younger. On the contrary, color that is too light can often highlight lines and wrinkles. A woman must consider the color of her eyes as well as the color of her skin when choosing a hair color.

→ *Eau de rose*, or rosewater, is an antioxidant. It cleans, clears, and protects color. Robin has products that incorporate the ingredient and they are wonderful, but one can mix *eau de rose* into shampoo and conditioner to get the desired effect. The correct ratio of shampoo or conditioner to rosewater is three parts to one.

→ Argan oil (from the nut of the argan tree, which is found primarily in Morocco), followed by an appropriate shampoo, can be a miracle remedy. Rich in omega-six fatty acids and antioxidants, it is used not only on hair, but also on skin. Because it is a "dry" oil, it adds remarkable shine and flexibility without making hair flat or greasy. Look for it in your health food store.

→ Lavender gives hair elasticity and shine.

→ Mother Nature knows what she's doing; no one should stray too far from her natural color.

→ For shine, fill a large bowl of cold water, add the juice of one lemon, and use the mixture for the final rinse. This makes all hair colors shine.

BLONDES, BRUNETTES, REDHEADS. . .

The most requested hair color is blonde; fortunately, it comes in almost infinite tones. Blonde hair has a long history: during the Renaissance, women covered their hair with a mélange of saffron and lemon juice and sat in the sun wearing hats with the tops cut out, leaving the brims to shade their faces and protect their porcelain skin, which was the revered complement to their soon-to-be blonde locks. Stylists often try subtly to steer their clients with darker complexions and dark eyes toward other colors, or toward caramel mixed into rich browns, for example.

"To me, blonde is easy," said Robin. "Brunette is gorgeous because it's like a little black dress. It's chic, it works, and it gives a beautiful effect. Red is not easy, but when it works it's extremely sexy."

Echoing the famous Coco Chanel quote "Look for the woman in the dress. If there is no woman, there is no dress," Robin said he never wants admirers of his work to say to a woman, "Your hair color is beautiful." Instead, he said he hoped they would compliment her by saying, "You look wonderful."

GRAY HAIR: AN "INTELLECTUAL" DECISION

As for gray, Robin said, "It takes guts to make that decision."

Rodolphe is famous for his artistic touch with gray hair. He refers to the decision to go gray as "intellectual." He added, "I think gray hair can be so modern and it shows enormous confidence. It gives a woman new freedom."

He continued, "It requires an attitude. It's part of

an emotional dress code. Going gray or white is another affirmation of femininity and, of course, deciding not to be a slave to your hair."

He has perfected a "microscopic" highlighting technique which he uses to take women whose hair is turning white or gray slowly into their new world of "salt and pepper," as he called it.

He has also been known to remove the color completely from a woman's hair in order to take it to the natural color of the gray roots. Sometimes the process takes more than two days to accomplish, because he does it almost hair by hair, and it's exhausting for him and the client. Diana, an American friend of mine who has lived most of her life in France, did precisely that with Rodolphe. She did not want to go through the grow-out phase, and she was bored and "frankly sick and tired of constant root touch-ups every three weeks," she told me.

"It was as if I got a 'get out of jail free' card. It was a nightmare with the constant root growth," Diana said. "Rodolphe did it over two days, about eight hours each time. I was terrified, but he kept passing by and telling me how gorgeous he finds young faces and white hair. He kept re-icing the cake when he saw I was getting nervous. The first day I left the salon, my hair was steel gray; the second day it was white, which it has been ever since. I can't tell you how happy I am."

I have one friend, Chantal, who has one of the most beautiful hair colors I have ever seen. She was a natural light blonde, and her hair turned white, but a white that mixed in with her blonde. It's gorgeous. And, it's natural.

All she does is wash it with a neutral shampoo, followed by another—with a violet hue to avoid yellowing—and the occasional deep conditioner. She's been stopped on the street by women asking the address of her colorist.

Both Robin and Rodolphe opt for modern, graphic haircuts for gray hair. To look young, gray hair must move and not be frizzy or wild. That's their opinion, and it's also the only way I've seen gray here. I'm sure many women don't agree. If gray is a gutsy, intellectual decision at the end of the day, perhaps the style is open for debate.

CARE AND MAINTENANCE

Like so many of the hairstylists and colorists with whom I spoke, Robin and Rodolphe are dismayed by the daily washing and product application that many women insist are important. Then, they lament, women wonder why their hair is flat or brassy. Those issues are the result of product buildup and the stripping of natural oils.

Natural oils in our hair, like those in our skin, are not our enemies.

Robin told me his celebrity clients often arrive for their color sessions with their hair covered with oil or with his lavender conditioner, which is out of this world (he gave me some), and pinned back into chignons in preparation for the process. "The oil unifies the porosity of the color," he explained.

Rodolphe also emphasized, "Always oil before color. It assures the color will 'take' beautifully."

News to me and my regular hairstylist. I tried it with Michelle; I explained I was experimenting for this chapter.

I'm convinced the color was richer and had more shine. She thought so, too.

While Robin and I were talking, he told me a couple of fun tricks for all of us. He said he learned the perfect way to towel-dry hair from one of his Moroccan clients. Let me try to explain: take a regular-sized bath towel and fold it three to four times. Next, bend forward (standing or sitting), toss your hair toward the floor, and quickly "whip" the towel from nape to ends, then from forehead to tips of the hair. Do this several times. I promise you, the result is quite surprising. Hair is damp, but you've built in volume, because air is whipped through it during the towel-dry process.

Both Rodolphe and Robin agreed my hair was in excellent condition. At least I'm doing something right.

Although the chic and *cher* salons of Christophe Robin and Rodolphe are two of the most coveted addresses in Paris for color and cater to some of the most famous and beautiful women in the world, their atmospheres are warm and welcoming. Any woman who walks through the doors of their salons is treated with the same care and kindness as the celebrities. The two men are absolutely adorable. When they talk about women, they are kind and respectful. They understand the special relationship women have with their hairstylists, and they both say they are flattered and touched by the confidence and generosity of the loyal coterie of women who can't live without them.

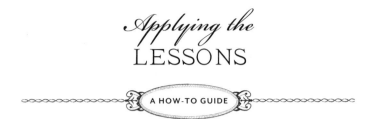

Applying the
LESSONS

A few things I learned from Rodolphe—who has Jodie Foster, Sophie Marceau, and Kate Hudson among his clients—and now (literally) apply:

⟡ Prior to using shampoos, which have been specifically chosen for the condition and color of one's hair, pour some "dry" oil—argan oil, for example—into the palms of the hands, rub them together to heat the oil, and apply it to the hair. Let it soak in for a few minutes, then wash.

⟡ Two shampoos a week are enough for most women, but women should shampoo twice during these bi-weekly washings.

⟡ Most women—count me among them—use way too much shampoo. All you need is a noisette, or hazelnut, in your hand. Add a little water, rub your hands together, and then spread the shampoo on the sides of your head and then the top. Same goes for conditioner. Less is more, and use it just on the lengths and ends.

⟡ My regular coiffeuse, Michelle, who does not have her own product line, tells me that it's more economical to buy professional hair products because they are more concentrated and we need less.

⟡ Blondes and women with white or gray hair should be using a second shampoo with a slight violet tint (a neutral product can be used for the first shampoo). We are not to use chamomile because it yellows our hair, heaven forbid. Qualifier: chamomile is fine for honey and caramel colors.

⟡ Hair masques are so important. Without exception, from the hairstylists to the stars to my Michelle, all recommended sleeping in deep conditioner once a month.

⟡ For color, bring a picture of yourself as a child to your next appointment. "I like to see photographs of women when they were children to see what their real hair colors once were. If possible, I would like to see several photos of the children as they age to observe the evolution of those colors," Rodolphe said.

⟡ For blondes, after a day in the sun, treat hair to three-quarters of a cup of argan oil and the juice of one lemon, whisked together like a vinaigrette and left on hair for thirty minutes. It boosts shine and color.

As you can imagine, a visit to either Christophe Robin or Rodolphe is an expensive experience, but they both have clients who save to have their hair colored by them.

One such client from a distant town in France had heard about Rodolphe. She saved for months, made her appointment, and took the train to Paris for her big day. When she left, Rodolphe gave her a card on which he had written the secret recipe for her hair color to give to her hairdresser in the town where she lives.

Délicatesse is a word the French often use to describe the kindness, the understanding, the gentle sensitivity that one shows another in situations that could be stressful or intimidating. Not to put too fine a point on it, because the subject here is hair after all, and *délicatesse* is usually applied to far more dramatic situations, but for me the word *did* apply when I saw the way clients were treated in some of the most exclusive hair salons in Paris.

In many cases, the women who walked through the doors of these emporiums were there for perhaps the first and last time. Some were slightly intimidated by the glamour and reputations beyond the threshold, and several were making enormous budgetary sacrifices for the experience. They came for help. Chances are the reasons for their appointments were far more complex than simply a masterful cut and perfect color. And, that's where the experts took over—part psychologists, part practitioners, part artists—as they spent the time, with *délicatesse*, to discover what would help make each woman happy, *bien dans sa peau.*

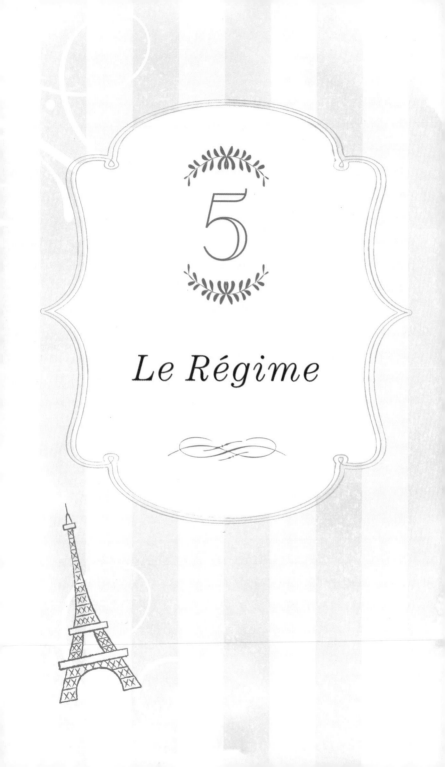

5

Le Régime

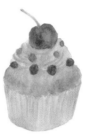

THE ART OF EATING WELL

The Marquise de Montespan, considered a great beauty and admired for her lush figure, was the longtime favorite of Louis XIV and mother of seven of his children. Bearing children inevitably led to what she—and others—considered a distressing weight gain. To quell her appetite, she supposedly drank vast amounts of vinegar. (One doctor told me this method probably works, but leaves you feeling rather unwell.)

Thanks to all the books and articles written on the subject, we're supposed to believe that Frenchwomen don't get fat. Basically that's true, they don't get *fat,* but they do from time to time need to lose a few kilos (there are 2.2 pounds per kilo for those of you needing to do the conversion). Without exception, every Frenchwoman I interviewed said being slender was a top priority and her major challenge.

I must say that made me feel better, knowing that it's not just genetic and supremely easy for them, while remaining such a struggle for others, including myself. Petite French girls learn early on how and what to eat to maintain their enviable figures throughout their lives. Habits start young, but that does not mean that women of a certain age cannot change their relationship with food. I have.

A HEALTHY APPROACH

France as a whole is committed to healthy eating. Written across the bottom of the television screen with every advertisement that could be interpreted as "snack" food—and that includes yogurt and applesauce—there is a reminder about consuming five vegetables and fruits each day.

Recently I saw a sweet television ad for baby food that showed a devoted mother spooning a classic fruit purée into her adorable child's mouth—to the evident delight of her *enfant*. A few seconds into the product advertisement, the following warning flashed across the bottom of the screen: "Teach your children not to snack between meals."

There's no escaping it.

From the time a child is weaned off the breast or the bottle, the beverage introduced at meals is water. One will not see tall glasses of icy cold milk at each child's place or gigantic bottles of soda in the center of the dinner table. French children drink water with their meals and, indeed, whenever they're thirsty, just like *maman*. French children also discover the differences among the flavors and textures of a vast variety of foods. Toddlers eat fennel and cabbage (or at least are introduced to them, as well as to other "exotic" foods). They understand, because they have yet to experience the contrary, that everything they eat does not have to be sweet.

They also understand early on, thanks to their mothers and grandmothers, that food is not the enemy. It's the grazing and overindulgence in thoughtless eating that are the enemy.

Little girls are not only learning lessons about eating well at table, but also about preparing food in the kitchen. By the age of eight or ten, many are capable of preparing apple tarts without adult assistance. The rituals that go into preparation, presentation, and eating are the ingredients that help place food in its proper context—pleasure and, as we all know, moderation.

A French family might finish an evening meal with a homemade fruit compote (no sugar added, of course) of apples and pears and/or some yogurt. Tarts, cakes, mousses, and crème brûlée are treats. They are consumed with great delight and anticipation once a week, no more. In fact, many nutritionists recommend fruit compotes in the evening. Not only do they provide a sweet finish to dinner, but at least one nutritionist told me that applesauce (*compote de pommes*) helps us sleep better.

The healthy relationship Frenchwomen have with food automatically leads them to a realistic quantity/quality approach to eating. For the most part, the French save cocktail hours and luscious desserts for exceptional, special occasions.

And they seem to know instinctively when to make a calorie splurge and when it's just not worth it.

THE FASHION CONNECTION

One afternoon, when I was on an undercover assignment for this chapter, I noticed that, as I was spooning whipped cream onto my syrupy thick, obscenely delicious hot chocolate *chez* Angelina—which serves what is arguably the best *chocolat chaud* in all of Paris—the Frenchwomen around me were sipping tea with paper-thin slices of lemon floating on the un-sugared surface. And they seemed to be enjoying themselves immensely.

"We're brought up in a culture where we have always been close to fashion and food. Furthermore, Frenchwomen are very competitive; they want to be the best at everything— lover, mother, cook, career woman—while all the time being stylish," dietician Claire Brosse-Dandrieux, told me. "And, let's be frank, to look good in your clothes you have to be relatively slim."

Another *ah-ha* moment: It's all about personal style, and vanity is a powerful appetite suppressant.

To conduct my research, I observed my friends during our lunches and at parties, spied on random Frenchwomen with those enviable figures when they were out at restaurants, and, of course, talked to experts in the know.

Frenchwomen judiciously watch their weight. They have a set weight point and from that number they allow themselves a two-to-three-kilo fluctuation for the holidays, special events, vacations, etc. There are myriad advantages to their way. They can wear the same clothes for years; it's better for their health; they are in control of their bodies, not the reverse, which is infinitely satisfying (mind over matter); and they are literally and figuratively more comfortable *dans leur peaux* ("in their skin", that famous French expression).

If that isn't sufficient incentive, Dr. Jean-Louis Sebagh, one of the world's leading plastic surgeons, pointed out that keeping one's weight within a reasonable range is one of the best anti-age treatments that exists. "Frenchwomen intrinsically understand," he said. "It's never a good idea for the face to be too gaunt with excessive dieting and exercise, or to be yo-yoing after a certain age. Too thin, and the face does not have the 'fat' cushion of youth. Too many major fluctuations and the face becomes flaccid. It cannot spring back into shape after a certain age. It's about balance, and that's something Frenchwomen apply to all aspects of their lives."

With few exceptions, my friends and the women I met while writing this book told me they are *gourmandes* at heart. Translation: they love to eat and might fleetingly consider larger proportions of their favorite foods if they didn't love some of their favorite clothes even more.

I once saw my friend Genevieve Guerlain swoon over a slice of chocolate cake at a large gala, and then take her fork and gently cut off a morsel that only went halfway up the tines. That was it. She didn't even take her bite off the end with all the icing. Yet she told me, eyes gleaming, "I adore chocolate cake."

Recently we lunched at her glorious apartment. She said on the phone the day before, "It's just the two of us. We'll have a girls' lunch. How does that sound?"

It sounded perfect to me. The meal included individual salads of vegetables and seafood, bread as one can find only in Paris, butter if one so wished (no one did), wine, and for dessert a tiny red-fruit crumble. For coffee we moved into the salon and there, right next to the tray, was a box of chocolates. We each had one.

For years, I was convinced all their talk about loving to eat was mostly *coquetterie*. There is, after all, something exceedingly sensuous about eating heartily—particularly at a dinner party or when dining *tête-à-tête* with a man—yet remaining slender. And Frenchwomen do eat heartily from time to time, but then it's right back on the wagon.

I'm certain it's the very fact that Frenchwomen truly love good food (and wine) that is responsible for their success with their weight control. Eating delicious and nutritious meals every day is the only real secret for getting and staying slim. Often as much care goes into choosing food as into its preparation. Elaborate meals are the exception; simple meals are the norm.

Now, like most Frenchwomen, I shop for fresh produce three times each week. The market is one of my favorite places, and over the years I've built up relationships with the vegetable men, one of whom chooses my artichokes—if the petals are closed, it means they're fresh—the cheese lady, who is generous with samples and knows the percentage of fat in every one of her *fromages*; the fish man (he throws in a few extra langoustines after he weighs our order); the young man who sells roasted chicken and always tries to speak English with me; the fruit man who chooses the melons for today and three days from now. He puts an X on the one for today. It's an adventure; it's part of what I love about living in France.

My friend Edith says she eats "efficiently." What she means is she will choose seasonal fruit over sugary confections (although if you put a coffee éclair from Lenôtre in front of her, all semblance of reason evaporates). She starts every meal with either a soup in winter or a salad sprinkled with wheat germ and bean sprouts, and she eats brown rice, never white. She is a vegetable, fruit, and fish fiend.

"I eat the best of what my body needs and, as a result, I have tons of energy," she said. That's true; it's exhausting just watching her. "I never think about my weight. I have never been on a diet. I have a three-tiered steamer and cook almost everything in it, so I'm not adding unnecessary calories, but then I'll sauté fresh mushrooms in olive oil to make the meal more interesting."

Alexandra Fourcade, internist and mother of three daughters between the ages of sixteen and twenty-six, says she, too, has never been on a diet. "Diets are passé," she proclaimed. "They are too mentally time-consuming. I don't even think about eating anymore. I know what's good for me and what isn't. My body tells me. I'm attuned to how I feel when I eat well, or less well. When I make exceptions for wine, champagne, or a dessert, it's a conscious decision and I enjoy every second.

"Alcohol," she and all the individuals I interviewed agreed, "is not conducive to beautiful skin." Another reason to imbibe with moderation.

When one of Dr. Fourcade's daughters was having problems with her weight, Dr. Fourcade took her to a nutritionist. She followed the regime and now eats like her mother and her sisters—no dieting necessary. "No nagging from her mother, either," Fourcade pointed out. "It was her decision and her responsibility."

Everyone I know tends to eat light dinners at home. In the summer, salads, fruits, and sometimes fish grilled on the barbeque, and in the winter, soups. Yogurt is very often the dessert of choice for every day. In the winter we make fruit compotes of apples and pears—without sugar, of course.

Because a French meal usually commences with a small appetizer, such as a salad or a simple soup, the brain has time to register the hungry/satisfied equation as we move slowly into

Vinaigrette

Combine two tablespoons of extra-virgin olive or cold-pressed, unfiltered canola (rapeseed) oil; one tablespoon water (the water replaces what would normally be a third measure of oil); one tablespoon vinegar or lemon juice; one tablespoon mustard; and fresh herbs. Whisk briskly. The mustard holds the oil and water mixture together. (All recipes for vinaigrette are three to one—my three are two measures of oil and one water, plus one measure of vinegar or lemon juice, which is to say a larger quantity can be made using the same formula.)

the main course. Time is built into a repast naturally. As we all know, the brain-stomach connection takes between twenty to thirty minutes.

FAIRE ATTENTION

Still, Frenchwomen, like the rest of us, sometimes need to *faire attention*, or "to pay attention," as they say, which translates into a *régime*. They, too, have turned to faddish food combinations and quick-trick diets. (You may recall the latest in that category was French, but it has now been rejected not only by women, but also by the medical community.) Some have asked their doctors for magic pills, but all they come away with these days are various herbal remedies, which at least give a psychological boost.

But, bottom line, there is no magical French pharmaceutical solution, a bullet *d'argent*, if you will. My internist told me, "There are two secrets: the decision and apples." *Pardonnez-moi*?

Both he and Claire Brosse-Dandrieux emphasized the fact that diets work only when we make sure we are never hungry, or, if we are, that we have an immediate, natural— "natural" means no processed foods allowed—solution to the problem within easy reach. The first line of defense for every Frenchwoman I know is hot tea. It gives us a minute to think before we are overcome by a rash, thoughtless desire to stuff something into our mouths.

My internist keeps several apples in his car at all times. My pal Françoise never leaves home without hard-boiled eggs on days she's not sure she will be able to get to "the right food," and my best friend, Anne-Françoise, always tucks a bag of almonds in her handbag. "You never know," she said.

Frenchwomen eat three meals a day, every day. That probably explains why a mid-afternoon snack, if they indulge in one at all, is minimal—as in, tea with a piece of fruit, two squares of dark chocolate, a yogurt (always plain, 2 percent, never fat-free, sometimes with fresh fruit), or a few almonds, for example. (Edith soaks her almonds in water so they sort of "sprout," which she claims make them more healthful and easier to digest.)

My research indicated that she is, once again, absolutely correct. Soaking almonds breaks down the fiber and makes them easier to digest. News to me. Among all the miracles associated with almonds is the fact that they are also supposed to be a "brain tonic," full of essential fats that boost memory and intelligence.

Among my friends and acquaintances, no one is skeletal. I've come to see them over the years as normal. It's true I live *near* Paris, but not *in* Paris, so I have a broader view of Frenchwomen and their figures. My eye has become accustomed to women who are slender, but not shockingly so. Let's remember, too: Inès de la Fressange, with her extra long, lean body, is the great French exception. Most Frenchwomen are of medium height and small boned.

MINDFUL EATING

I recently met a well-known French doctor, Denis Lamboley, who specializes in nutrition and has, for me at least, some fresh approaches to the challenge of weight loss and life-long maintenance.

Dr. Lamboley urges his patients to come to terms with the stresses and emotions that lead them to food as a panacea. "Imagine you are confronted with a menace," he said. "What do you do? You decide how to escape from that threat. You think; you act. That is crucial, not only in the weight-loss process, but also more importantly in life-long maintenance. Think before you act. Practice mindfulness."

Mindfulness refers to being completely in touch with the present moment while at the same time not judging the thought one is holding, or the experience one is having. The term, as you may know, comes from Eastern spiritual and religious traditions like Zen Buddhism, and Dr. Lamboley encourages his patients to use it when addressing stress, emotion, and, in the case of food, temptation. He emphasizes that once we step back from a situation and make a decision, we accept and move on. He dislikes the idea of guilt associated with food and promises that if one is mindful about decisions, guilt will evaporate.

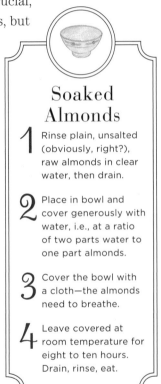

Soaked Almonds

1 Rinse plain, unsalted (obviously, right?), raw almonds in clear water, then drain.

2 Place in bowl and cover generously with water, i.e., at a ratio of two parts water to one part almonds.

3 Cover the bowl with a cloth—the almonds need to breathe.

4 Leave covered at room temperature for eight to ten hours. Drain, rinse, eat.

He pointed out that there are only two reasons to eat: hunger and pleasure. That's my new mantra – very French indeed. He also said that if we want to eat something purely for pleasure and we make a conscious decision to go ahead and eat those two quarter-size *macarons*, we should do so "and enjoy them. Don't feel guilty, not for one second."

Claire said something similar regarding the siren song we all know so well: chocolate, chocolate, chocolate. You're familiar with those moments when that's all you can think about, your sole fantasy. What should you do?

"Go for it," she said. "If you don't, you'll have a no- or low-fat yogurt, and you'll still be thinking about chocolate, so you'll have another yogurt, and you'll still be thinking about chocolate. Next you'll have a piece of fruit. And then what? You want chocolate! At this point, you'll break down and have the chocolate, but you'll have downed two yogurts and a peach and you weren't satisfied. You wanted chocolate; you should have had chocolate."

As anyone who has read anything on the subject knows, the chocolate of choice should be dark, at least 70 percent cocoa, eaten slowly and savored, maybe with a cup of tea to prolong the enjoyment.

"It must be eaten without guilt," Claire said emphatically. "When it comes to foods like chocolate, desire has nothing to do with hunger. You cannot make substitutes for desires. They're psychological, not physiological, and life is entirely too short to deny pleasure."

FOOD AS FÊTE

Years ago I read a survey wherein Frenchwomen and American women were asked the question "What is the first thing that comes into your mind when you think of chocolate cake?"

The Frenchwomen responded, "fête," while the Americans said, "sinful." One clearly sees the difference in mindsets. Furthermore, by definition "fête" means an exception, a celebration.

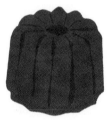

An impulse lasts for twelve minutes. Elyane Lèbre, an associate of Dr. Lamboley's who creates many of the recipes he likes, explained this to me as we sat on the terrace of the Royal Monceau hotel, drinking iced coffee and enjoying two quarter-sized *macarons* each. She suggested that we can overcome an impulse by immediately doing something for twelve minutes, like polishing our nails, for example, or making a phone call. Mindfulness helps us identify the menace and keeps us in the moment; then we decide.

Recently I met with Dr. France Aubry, internist, nutritionist, author, and woman of a certain age. "A *régime* is not punishment," Dr. Aubry said. "It must be constructed in a way that makes it possible to stay on it until one's goal weight is achieved and then live and eat normally with intelligence." Like every doctor and dietician I've met, Dr. Aubry also counsels her patients to be realistic about the numbers on the scale.

A SENSIBLE FRENCH *REGIME*

A SAMPLE WEEK

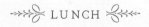

⟶⟶☙ BREAKFAST ☙⟵⟵

Fresh lemon juice in a tall glass of room-temperature water (too hot and it destroys the vitamin C), one kiwi, two slices of whole-wheat toast lightly swiped with real butter, one or two eggs or two yogurts (4.4 ounces or 125 grams each) made from 2-percent milk, and a very large *café au lait*. The milk is, again, 2-percent.

* You can vary this, keeping the elements of protein, fat, fruit, hot beverage. Breakfast is the same on regular days, free days, and Top Model days.

⟶⟶☙ LUNCH ☙⟵⟵

One of the following: a slice of ham with the fat trimmed away, the white meat of chicken or turkey, water-packed tuna, or any other fish; a salad with a small serving of vinaigrette (see recipe page 124); one piece of fruit except bananas, grapes, or dried fruit.

You can see that a chef's salad can be made with these ingredients.

TOP MODEL DIET LUNCH (three days per week): seven ounces (200 grams) of fish or white-meat chicken or 5.3 ounces (150 grams) of meat. A 5-ounce lean hamburger is a nice size portion. Two 4.4-ounce yogurts or 7 ounces of *fromage blanc*, which is probably hard to find in the U.S., unfortunately.

⟶⟶☙ DINNER ☙⟵⟵

Vegetable soup, fish or white meat, cooked green vegetable, and one yogurt or one fruit.

TOP MODEL DIET DINNER: Vegetable soup or 14 to 17 ounces of cooked green vegetables with one tea-spoon of olive oil. For dessert, two baked apples or a fruit compote, both without sugar, of course.

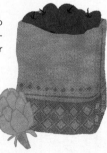

**Important: *The Top Model Diet meals are to be eaten on the same day. The protein lunch staves off hunger; the light dinner finishes the day with the vitamins we need to stay healthy. No wine on these days.*

Specifically, this is why her *régime* is so successful and no doubt the reason why she is famous in France. Her *régime* is basically as follows: No, favorite foods are not put on hold until the maintenance phase. She allows two "free" meals per week—one lunch, one dinner—and that could mean, for example, *boeuf Bourguignon* and potatoes, wine, and an unsweetened fruit dessert (she suggests pineapple). If, in one of those meals, fish is substituted for the meat, dessert can be a chocolate éclair.

Three days a week feature her Top Model Diet within the diet, wherein breakfast remains the same, lunch is all protein, and dinner is either a vegetable potage with a compote of fruit or cooked green vegetables (quantity: four hundred to five hundred grams) with a teaspoon of olive oil, and for dessert a fruit compote or two baked apples.

She allows two glasses of wine per day. I never drink two glasses of wine a day, but the idea that the possibility is out there is appealing in the sense that she understands that wine offers pleasure.

This is the easiest diet I've ever encountered, and three of my French friends who have tried it agree. The Top Model Diet is also a great way to get back on track after holidays, copious dinner parties, or any overindulging.

Dr. Aubry prescribed a magic—and no, I'm not exaggerating—plant-based pill, Madécassol, that was originally formulated as a natural circulation aid, which she discovered has a beneficial side effect as a diuretic that helps reduce cellulite. When I went to the pharmacy to have my prescription filled, the pharmacist assured me that it would work. And it does!

She also gives her patients a prescription for massages by a physical therapist to help rid the body of water and waste, cellulite again. I almost hate to tell you this, but here goes: these sessions are covered by the French socialized healthcare system. I said to Dr. Aubry, "*Vive la France.*" She said, "*N'est-ce pas?*" The massages are brilliant and literally make a measurable difference, as with a tape measure. However, since I'm doing hands-on research for this chapter, I must tell you they are not fun, although Frenchwomen are addicted to them. Massage is definitely an oxymoron in this case. Never do the therapist's hands touch the body. Instead, the patient slips into a neck-to-ankle body stocking—no underwear allowed—and a machine is used to knead the skin. Unfortunately, while kneading, the contraption also sucks and pinches the skin. The thing has several speeds, and the therapist can (and does) apply serious pressure to her task. The experience can best be described as an attack by an industrial vacuum cleaner on steroids.

The procedure must be followed by copious water consumption to flush out the cellulite. Yes, it works. It's not a miracle, but it does help contour the body and it aids the draining process. Frenchwomen like accompaniments to their *régimes*, which can also include hammams, steam baths, and real-deal massages at beauty institutes and spas.

Q & A
WITH DR. AUBRY

Q Some of my friends and I like to drink our wine before dinner; it's more fun (read: buzz). Is that acceptable? And, may I please chose white wine if the spirit moves me?

A You may drink wine before dinner, but eat dinner quickly thereafter. You want the alcohol to be digested with your meal. And, yes, you may drink white wine, although I prefer red. Remember, though, white could make you nervous.

Q What if one is really, really hungry at four or five p.m. and is tempted to make a regrettable decision in front of a gooey empty-calorie temptation?

A Eat a piece of fruit, have some tea, or fruit and a yogurt or a glass of tomato juice or V-8. Yes, you can have a small handful of almonds.

Q What do you think of herbal tea before bed?

A Love it.

Q Legumes, i.e., lentils, etc. Where do you stand?

A Love them. A small bowl can be eaten with fish or eggs, but not meat on the regular days.

Q Chocolate?

A After a meal, dark, of course, and in moderation.

Q What about cheese? We live in France, after all.

A Soft cheeses only, such as Camembert, Brie, chèvres (goat cheeses), etc. Not every day—occasionally—and then no dessert.

Q Water?

A Not enough is not good, too much is an error. We should consume one and a half liters of liquid daily. Too much leads to retention, not enough and the entire body suffers—inside and out. I recommend one liter of water. We get the rest of the liquids we need from other beverages during the day. (Ed. note [that's me]: All my girlfriends drink a minimum of one and a half liters of water per day.)

Q We all know you'll say no to sugar, but for heaven's sake, how about a little honey, agave, or xylitol (a natural, very sweet "sugar" made from the bark of birch trees) occasionally, on a yogurt maybe?

A Fine, but only one teaspoon. And don't abuse the privilege.

Q What's your stand on detoxing?

A I think it's great, but only one day per week. I suggest my patients do their detoxes with a vegetable bouillon, herbal tea with a teaspoon of honey, and a fruit compote. This is wonderful for the complexion as well.

Now for a review of what Frenchwomen know about maintaining their figures and a healthy attitude toward food:

- **ADD A SOUP OR SALAD.** Some experts say that by adding a first course to every meal, we cut as many as 20 percent of the total calories from lunches and dinners. Vegetable soup is a marvel!

- **SIT DOWN WHEN YOU EAT.** I have never seen a Frenchwoman eat standing up in her kitchen—or anywhere else for that matter. Yes, you know this, but it eclipses mindfulness, and mindfulness is our new way to live.

- **EAT WITH PLEASURE AT EVERY MEAL.** Enjoy your food.

- **HAVE CHOCOLATE WITHOUT REMORSE,** when you want it, but make it dark and in small amounts. The hours between four and six p.m. are the best times to eat chocolate, said Dr. Lamboley. Dr. Aubry prefers after a meal. (I think about it, i.e., am mindful, and then I eat it no matter what time of day. But, I only eat a small portion. Before I moved to France, I had no idea a candy bar could be savored and saved.)

- **READ LABELS.** "If something has more than five ingredients, it's probably not good for us," Elyane Lèbre said.

- **RUSH RIGHT OUT AND BUY A STEAMER.** All my friends have them; Edith's has three tiers. It's a flavorful way to cook and to discover the essence of foods.

- **ON THE OUTSIDE CHANCE YOU DO NOT OWN A BLENDER, YOU'LL WANT ONE** for soups and smoothies. The French have taken to smoothies with a collective passion.

- **LISTEN TO YOUR BODY.** A Frenchwoman stops at or before the point of feeling full during a meal, regardless of whether there is still food on her plate.

You will be surprised by how easy it is. Once you have adopted the French way of celebrating both food *and* figure, you will find it becomes a remarkably pleasurable and simple way to live.

6

Exercise?
Bien Sûr!

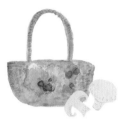

LA *FEMME FRANÇAISE* FORMULA:
FITNESS FOR THE FUN OF IT

While I'm teaching English conversation on Friday mornings, in a room next to ours, women are reaching for the sky in their stretching classes, and down the hall another group of women are throwing themselves into Pilates (pronounced *Pee-lots* or *Pee-lot*, depending upon whether the women employ the silent French *s*). Two acquaintances are doing tai chi. Many other Frenchwomen I know have signed up for some form of yoga.

As for my *aquagym* classes, they are so popular that postulants are turned away. This year I dragged myself out of bed at eight a.m. on a Saturday (!) to stand in line for two hours, just to get on the list. For my three hundred sixty euros per year, I have the possibility of attending seven *aquagym* classes each week. (One year I actually did go seven times a week.)

What do all these exercise activities have in common? The vast majority of participants are Frenchwomen of a certain age. They are exercising for a variety of reasons. Some wish to boost their metabolisms as menopause sets in. Some wish to keep their bodies feeling young, their movements fluid.

In my *aquagym* class, women range in age from their twenties (some are new mothers), to one woman who likes to boast, as well she should, that she is eighty-three. She said it helps her arthritis, and seeing her gallivant in and out of the pool, it's clear her water therapy is working. She often rides her bicycle to the pool.

An acquaintance who recently celebrated her seventieth birthday told me her three weekly exercise classes—stretching, yoga, and tai chi—keep her arthritis at bay and allow her to move, walk, and bicycle with the same ease she did when she was in her thirties. I've seen her walking in town—she does all of her market shopping on foot with a large basket slung over her arm—and she moves like a young woman, quickly and lithely.

One of my students, in her early forties, wears her bathing suit under her clothes and dashes off to the indoor pool next door the minute the class is finished to do laps before she has lunch.

All of this goes to show that Frenchwomen *do* exercise and are doing so in increasing numbers. Do not believe all the nonsense you've heard and read claiming Frenchwomen of a certain age do not exercise. Believe me, they do. We're exercising together.

Anne Breton, a classically trained dancer and instructor of the above-mentioned nonaquatic exercise class, plus dance and fitness courses, told me the other day that she also gives personal training lessons as a result of the growing demand from her students, particularly women of a certain age, who know the one-on-one attention will help them exercise correctly and thus more efficiently. I asked her the age range of her class participants and her private students, "From their thirties to seventy-plus," she said. "Some women attend three times a week, others only once. It often depends upon whether they work or not. I've seen an explosion in gym exercising in the last ten years. I think women realize that to stay healthy and feel youthful, i.e., to have bodies that move with ease, they have to exercise."

Breton has been teaching various forms of exercise, as well as jazz and ballet, for twenty-six years. Her basic class is a tough sixty minutes, she concedes, and includes squats, stretching, and concentration on abdominals, derriere, and arms, and it finishes with relaxing stretching. "Gradually, as the class progresses, I'll add weights and elastics," she said. She also teaches step classes.

She noted that her classes are not a lark. "I've seen exercise sessions where women chat, exchange recipes, talk about whatever, but not in my classes. We're there to work and we concentrate on the exercises," she said. "It is fun, though," she assured me.

Although Breton doesn't teach Pilates, she is a huge fan of the discipline. "It's simply a wonderful way to align the body, stretch, and move. It defies age."

She said in the new exercise explosion she has witnessed, she sees women taking up jogging in increasing numbers. "And it's not only very young women," she said. "Women in their forties and fifties are jogging these days." Breton is small-boned and has, as one would imagine, considering she exercises twenty-eight hours a week (not counting working with her personal-training clients), an enviable figure. She said she does not diet, but eats properly. "Let's put it this way though; I don't deprive myself, ever."

When I watch her acolytes file into the gym, I see women of normal builds, some slim, others less so—in fact a few are *un peu ronde*. They are basically a microcosm of the women I see every day. Anne explains to her pupils that exercise can sculpt the body, build muscle, and keep the joints moving comfortably, but "if you want to lose weight, you have to cut calories." She said that she has so much muscle that she weighs considerably more than the charts suggest for her height. "I have to keep explaining that phenomenon to women."

Our conversation flowed from muscle to cellulite, where she had another no-hesitation response: "Women have cellulite. I have cellulite." I find that hard to believe, but she swears it's true. It doesn't bother her, because it's minimal, but she uses herself as an example to explain to women that chances are they, too, will have some.

Rarely does a month go by that most women's magazines don't have articles on exercise. These types of stories were practically nonexistent when we first moved to France.

Health clubs offering various degrees of refinement and luxury are popping up all over the country. Some are simple, but each usually includes a pool large enough for *aquagym* classes, if not for serious laps, exercise classes, gyms with instructors and basic equipment, and often the little extra Frenchwomen of all ages adore—a *hammam*.

In Paris, not surprisingly, one can find breathtakingly beautiful spas that offer the hard-core with the *haut chic*. In the past several years, the best hotels have been adding more and more sumptuous exercise and pampering amenities. After a vigorous workout, you can partake of superb treatments that are so skillfully executed that you start wishing you could live there. At least one, where I spent an unforgettable day, will soon have an entire wellness program that will include all of the above, plus personalized diet recommendations. I was told some such regimens may have nothing to do with weight loss, but rather will be designed for well-being and even complete anti-age purposes—that goes for both exercise and food recommendations.

One need not be staying at a hotel, either. France, to my knowledge at least, in this domain, as in so many others, has a unique approach to the quality of life of its citizens. Towns and villages, no matter their size, offer classes at reasonable prices, and inhabitants can sign up for myriad offerings to enrich their lives. Among the options available in the town where I teach my English conversation classes are outings with experts to museums (a bus picks everyone up at the town hall, drives them into Paris for the day, and returns at six p.m.); painting classes of all types for all ages; computer lessons on several levels; piano lessons; book clubs; and also a variety of dance and exercise programs. The town has a population of 3,400 and a swimming pool where a menu of lessons and exercise classes is available.

Women of a certain age are enthusiastic participants. One of my students, in her sixties, leaves her computer class, crosses the vestibule to English, and ninety minutes later heads over to the pool.

Many of the classes, the exercise classes in particular, are *à la carte,* and there are family discounts, senior discounts, and the possibility of signing up for exercise classes and the pool by the hour according to one's schedule and budget. There are also evening classes, convenient for those who work during the day.

While selecting white peaches at my favorite market recently, I realized I was standing next to a friend from my *aquagym* class whom I hadn't seen in nearly a year. After the initial how-are-yous, we started talking about exercise. Marie, who is in her seventies, told me she had moved to Versailles and is now doing her *aquagym* there.

"Here's the best part," she said. "They have those water bikes. I'm starting slowly, but they're incredible. I never would have imagined riding a bicycle submerged in a swimming pool."

She started to encourage me to join her. "We can have lunch after," she added to sweeten the deal. I'm tempted.

Versailles is about thirty minutes from our house, whereas my usual, less sophisticated, though excellent, *aquagym* classes are a five minute door-to-door drive. If I were really serious, I would make the fifteen-minute bike ride.

In another town, Houdan, about twenty minutes from us in the other direction, a new state-of-the art gym, which has aquabikes, was opened by the municipality. My friend Michelle, forty-three, told me you must call in advance to reserve the *velos* for twenty-minute supervised lessons. "If you're three minutes late, you lose your place," she said. "The demand is unbelievable."

Even the beyond-exclusive Polo Club (referred to simply as "Le Polo"—everyone understands the reference), which was founded in 1892 by the Viscount de La Rochefoucauld in Paris, has, to the chagrin of many members, put bicycles in its swimming pool. "We go there to do our laps," one member told me. "The bicycles are annoying."

It's true, I think, that Frenchwomen of a certain age in particular view exercising differently from the way we do. They tend not to be advocates of "no pain, no gain." I've always considered Frenchwomen to be rather sportif and that inclination, combined with the way they naturally tend to incorporate walking and bicycling into their lives, definitely gives them "no pain, all gain" benefits.

They also prefer an element of fun. It makes my heart flip-flop in fear when I see women of a certain age (well, any age, actually) weaving through Paris traffic, skirts flying and heads unprotected by helmets, but they look carefree and content, as if they're having the time of their lives.

On the strictly sportif side, tennis is big, golf is growing apace in popularity, and, in our corner of the world, horseback riding is huge. Need I add that this is golf without golf carts? Both sports are entertaining, social, and calorie-burning. When I mention golf carts to French friends, they are mystified. They say they thought they were out there for exercise. Three friends are taking golf lessons, and one is participating in tournaments at the behest of her husband.

"I hate the competitive aspect because I'm such a terrible player, but I'm thinking that theoretically it should help my game," she said with a sort of withering sigh. "I keep reminding myself how good the fresh air is for me."

After a certain age, most Frenchwomen turn to doubles on the tennis court—mixed doubles when possible. It's more fun and involves less running, and it's so exceedingly French to find a way to double one's pleasure. The fact that everyone prefers *mixed* doubles clearly heightens the fun factor. "It's amazing how my husband and I can be super-competitive against our friends while laughing at the same time," an acquaintance told me. "We feel like children again. It definitely doesn't feel like exercise, but it definitely feels good."

Most women my age, and on either side of my decade, like to take their exercise with a refreshing dose of fresh air whenever possible. Many see folly in bicycling in a gym, even though they're willing to get down on the floor with their mats and work up a slight sweat. They don't rule out inside workouts, but they seem to have a visceral need for simultaneous communion with nature. It has been suggested that this desire is a natural and logical extension of France's agricultural heritage. Deep breaths of country air, they believe, keep one young and energetic. They also extol the antidepressant virtues of communing with nature.

I have never been to a large Sunday lunch in the country that was not followed by a long walk after *café*.

Every weekend, near the Rambouillet forest where we live, families bicycle on the paths winding through one of the most beautiful hunting reserves of the former French kings. Grandmothers and mothers lead the way with a trail of offspring of various ages following behind like ducklings.

Frenchwomen not only want their children to eat fresh fruits and vegetables every day, but they also want them to get fresh air as often as possible. *Aeration* is part of the French esthetic, another aspect of taking good care of oneself. An added incentive for the promenades is the possibility, in the summer, of picking wild blackberries or, in the fall and winter, mushrooms. These pastimes have been part of family weekends for generations.

Mushroom-picking is revered in the French country-side. (And every French pharmacy offers the free service of telling its customers whether the *champignons* in their baskets are edible or poisonous.) Mush-room aficionados have their secret corners in the forest where, for years, they have been plucking their finds from beneath the cover of dead leaves and moss. Most will never divulge their locations, but they do share their

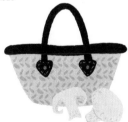

harvests. One great friend makes at least four or five *cèpe* deliveries to me every year. Where she finds the mushrooms is her best-kept secret. I'm perfectly happy with our arrangement.

Apart from the exercise built into daily lifestyles, family sports-related vacations are part of the culture. That means *sports d'hiver*, or winter sports (read: skiing), and summers planned around outdoor activities. Most French children are taken to the slopes when they can barely walk. My daughter went with friends to their chalet, and her school offered ski excursions. My husband's niece, a doctor in her early fifties, takes two ski vacations, one in March, the other in December, with her husband and three daughters. In the summer they rent a house near Biarritz, where the entire family windsurfs. (On the weekends she also bicycles in the country, and twice a week after work she does laps in an Olympic pool near her house in Neuilly.)

Some families vacation every year in Brittany because they believe swimming in the ocean and breathing in the ions from the region guard against colds and flu for the entire year. My husband believes this to be true and claims that's one of the major reasons his family had a house only yards from the Atlantic when he was a child. He told me that his mother insisted on summer vacations in Brittany for that very reason. Like thousands of mothers and grandmothers today, she believed the Brittany sea air was the secret to keeping children cold- and flu-free throughout the school year.

My friend Edith has concocted her own exercise formula, which consists of daily swimming (in the spring, summer, and fall in the pool of her country house) followed by a sauna (she also has a sauna), bicycling, but not in Paris ("I'll ride my bike in the country, but I'm too terrified to take it out in Paris," she admitted), winter vacations on the slopes, and a five-day-a-week workout with Jane Fonda. She then tucks into her two pieces of six-grain toast with honey, a soy yogurt (she doesn't eat cow's milk products), green tea, and a handful of almonds she's previously soaked overnight in water to remove their skins. When she's in Paris, she walks everywhere and only takes the Metro when absolutely necessary.

Edith is one of the worst let's-suit-up-and-go-for-a-walk, post–Sunday lunch offenders. Rain or shine, snow or slush, wind or sleet—nothing discourages her from staunchly heading out to seek fresh air, no matter the meteorological conditions. When friends protest, she produces slickers, raincoats, hats, gloves, scarves, socks, and even boots in various sizes. A boot is too big? "Here, put on another pair of socks." In other words, no excuses. Upon 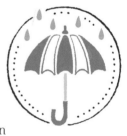 our return, she rewards us with tea, one oatmeal cookie each, and maybe, just maybe, two squares of dark chocolate, at least 70 percent cocoa.

Recently, I saw another one of those bottom-of-the-screen warnings pop up on the television screen. This was a new one for me. I'm quite familiar with the ones that caution against careless eating between meals and harp on five fruits and vegetables daily. This one said, "*Bouger!*" Or "Move!"

It's not the most sophisticated website out there in its design elements, but you might enjoy clicking over to www.mangerbouger.fr (eat/move), where you can get an idea of how the French think about eating and exercise. A special section titled "50 Ans et Plus," which means "50 and Over," is particularly interesting. You do not need to be fluent in the language—you'll definitely understand the message and the intention.

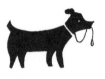

We can learn a great deal from the French practice of incorporating daily movement into our lives. When I walk with my dogs in the fields behind our house, wild berries are everywhere. My joy on these sojourns comes from the glee with which the dogs frolic in freedom, and from the fact that I return home with a basket of blackberries. When it's not berry season, I pick up kindling for the fireplace, some of which the dogs can carry. I'm an enthusiastic multitasker. The excursion is exercise without feeling like exercise, very French.

The
DRESS CODE

Even when they're dressed for ease of movement, Frenchwomen want some fit. Shapeless just doesn't do it for them.

The Frenchwomen I see in exercise classes wear some combination of the following: leggings, yoga pants with a clean-cut straight shape, T-shirts or tank tops, and some form of sports shoe. Usually a Frenchwoman will put a cardigan of some sort over her well-fitting, never-so-huge-she-drowns-in-it shirt.

Occasionally a woman will wear sweatpants, or "joggings," as the French call them, but the difference is, they fit. They are not baggy. They're slightly loose; they are not worn as camouflage gear.

As with their wardrobes, Frenchwomen do not opt for pastels or bright in-your-face colors in the gym or while jogging. They prefer navy, black, and gray. A white T-shirt or tank top can be part of the ensemble. No one wears message T-shirts.

N.B.: *No item of apparel that qualifies as a member of the sweatsuit family ever makes an appearance as alternative streetwear. Nor do gym or running shoes, for that matter. Frenchwomen get dressed to go out.*

7

Confronting
the Closet
Conundrum

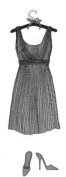

STAKING OUT NEUTRAL TERRITORY

Ah, the beauty of understatement trumping hyperbole. It took years to decipher the riddle. You know the one: Why is it that Frenchwomen of a certain age seem always to appear chic, feminine, confident, and-comfortable in their own skin?

What's so different about their wardrobes? Theoretically, we have equal access to most of the same offerings, but somehow we don't seem to pull them together to create the same naturally nonchalant effect. Why is that?

The clues were there all along, hiding in plain view, but like most investigators before me, I hadn't gotten beyond the exceedingly annoying *je ne sais quoi* explanation everyone used as a disappointing fallback. How in the world can we apply "an inexplicable something" to our wardrobe and well-being?

Then came the epiphany, the ah-ha moment: Frenchwomen like to be looked at.

Never mind the syntax; that's what an extremely elegant Frenchwoman of a certain age explained to me recently.

We met briefly while I was deep in conversation with a Frenchman of many interesting opinions on the subject of Frenchwomen and the pleasure they take in looking stylish, the way they "dress the part" for their own amusement and the entertainment of others.

Most of us are, most of the time, slightly uncomfortable with being observed. We like to be admired on many levels, including for our style choices, but we're not really "out there" on the metaphorical stage for appraisal. Frenchwomen are. They know that they are going to be observed, they are comfortable with that fact, and they prepare for it accordingly.

Some non-Frenchwomen (am I speaking to you?) imagine they're invisible if they venture out in sweats, shapeless message T-shirts, no makeup, and ponytails, but nothing could be farther from the truth. We're giving ourselves a bad reputation in the neighborhood, the grocery store, the mall, on vacation, *chez nous*, wherever. Getting dressed and getting out there garners respect and conveys self-confidence.

In conversations, interviews, and first meetings, we choose our words to convey our feelings, reveal various aspects of our personalities, our intellects, our moods. Therefore, never let it be said that our clothes do not speak to our intentions. Fashion is not trivial; it is an irrevocable part of who we are. We can construct "instant messaging" with our wardrobe choices.

I don't care if I never meet or see the same people on the street. My reputation is important to me, and I feel, as an American living abroad, that I have a patriotic obligation to uphold certain vestment standards.

JUST ADD ATTITUDE

No doubt you're thinking, "Great. I accept the concept, but how do I dress it up? How do those Frenchwomen of a certain age do it?"

Apart from my own observations, I asked them. Go to the source, I always say.

The foolproof French recipe for conquering now and forever that chronic, panic-provoking, I-have-nothing-to-wear scenario starts with a few basic, though intangible, ingredients.

A soupçon of attitude is essential. It starts with self-awareness—the body-mind connection.

Know thyself. As every Frenchwoman instinctively understands, unless you honestly assess and accordingly dress your body, great style is unattainable. The single, simple secret to timeless and ageless chic is to "know first who you are; and then adorn yourself accordingly" (Epictetus).

Then stand up straight.

The combination reflects an insouciant confidence, which is the way Frenchwomen wear their clothes. And since most of us know how to stand up straight, we can always feign the rest.

A major reason Frenchwomen of a certain age often appear younger than their years is the way they move. They have terrific posture—standing and sitting—and unless a Frenchwoman is strolling with a man or gossiping with her best friend, she tends to lope rather than walk down the street. She strides with shoulders back, head up, hair free, a slight swing of the arm not attached to a great bag, and her steps are long and purposeful. One has the impression she is on her way to an adventure.

Need I add that her posture and purposeful strides make her clothes look smart and stylish?

Factor in Frenchwomen's fixation on appearing ever *naturel,* and you've got the major components. A French-woman of a certain age will tell you she spent "absolutely no time" getting made up and dressing. She'll claim from the minute she rolled out of bed, slipped into the shower, applied her makeup and donned her apparel, total time: thirty minutes. She will never admit to fussing and buffing, and certainly not to indecision before her closet. I believe her, except maybe for the timeline, although I have a very good friend who pulls off the thirty-minute miracle every day. I stayed with her and her husband in their house in the South of France and saw her in action. She met the dead-line with a couple of minutes to spare, and she used those minutes to search for her sunglasses.

RETHINKING, REJECTING, RECASTING

By midlife, Frenchwomen know themselves so well that dressing with style is a reflex. They have found their best colors and cuts, and with only a few adjustments and a hand-ful of beloved items—the minis they collected in the 1970s, the transparent tops they flaunted through their thirties, the Azzedine Alaia dresses they can no longer *squeeeeeze* into— handed off to their daughters, nieces, and grand-daughters, they dress the way they've always dressed. That's what makes them appear young. They know the difference between the sublime and the ridiculous, which is not always the case with women who *try* to look young. Frenchwomen look great for their age naturally, seemingly effortlessly.

They wear many of their investment pieces for de-cades. But, let's be frank. There is another reason why they can continue to wear their clothes for many years: give or take two to four kilos, even with a slightly different distri-bution of their weight, the clothes still fit. When necessary, slight adjustments are made by their beloved seamstresses. That's another advantage of good clothes; they usually have some wiggle room built into the seams and hems.

Among the favorites that stay in the closet for the duration, one often finds a YSL black-leather pencil skirt (or maybe a similar, more budget friendly version from agnès b., for example); peasant blouses for summer; coats, all sorts of coats; ageless little black dresses. Favorites depend upon each woman. If she's very lucky, maybe she owns a Chanel suit. Chances are these days she wouldn't dream of wearing it all of a whole. She would wear the skirt with a turtleneck, a white shirt, and some hip accessories. Her leather jacket has moved away from tough toward feminine, but it does not move out of the wardrobe entirely and it works wonders with the Chanel skirt. As for the Chanel jacket, it *is* a cardigan after all. What can't one wear with a cardigan? Jeans, leather skirt, satin evening trousers ... You get the idea.

The leather skirt, which she may have saved for a year to buy, is never coupled with the leather jacket. Instead, it works well with whatever strikes one's fancy—it's a classic, after all. The peasant blouse is no longer worn as a "costume" with a peasant skirt, but looks fresh with white jeans. A creamy soft-leather jacket becomes an unexpected "rock 'n' roll" detail (as Frenchwomen like to say) when teamed with a gray flannel skirt and a white shirt or turtleneck sweater. A collection of well-cut T-shirts is essential, as are cashmere turtlenecks and V-necks, and a few crisp, white *chemises*.

As Karl Lagerfeld said, "Reinvent new combinations of what you already own. Improvise. Become more creative. Not because you have to, but because you want to. Evolution is the secret for the next step."

Frenchwomen of a certain age "recast" their favorite pieces. Their creativity in mixing the old with the new or the old with the old in new ways is a lesson in eternally evolving elegance.

Take the ever-flattering peasant skirt, for example. A Frenchwoman of a certain age would couple it with a T-shirt or a shirt, adding a cummerbund improvised out of a scarf, a wide belt, or even a ribbon to mark the waist. Espadrilles or sandals finish the outfit for a grown-up. Actually, it's an outfit for any age.

I have a great friend who has been wearing the same Yves Saint Laurent ankle-grazing fuchsia cotton "twirly skirt," as my daughter used to say when she was small, for as long as I've known her, which is approaching thirty years. One summer I decided to count how many different ways she put it together. She made it work for Paris, the country, shopping, weddings, Sunday lunches in the garden, her grandson's baptism, plus casual and more chichi dinner parties. I actually took notes about what she paired it with, just for fun:

1) *Large Hermès scarf as a halter.*
2) *White poplin shirt, the tails tied at the waist.*
3) *White cotton piqué Spencer jacket.*
4) *Pale pink men's oxford button-down shirt, tucked in, with a large black belt.*
5) *Multicolored silk striped vest—the fuchsia was repeated in one of the stripes.*
6) *Black silk moiré vest.*
7) *A pretty Pucci blouse she has owned forever.*
8) *Wide pink-and-white-striped poplin shirt, tucked in with a wide navy grosgrain ribbon at the waist.*
9) *White sleeveless blouse, cut like a halter.*
10) *Polo shirts.*
11) *Navy linen Spencer.*
12) *A white ribbed Marcel.*
13) *An embroidered peasant blouse.*
14) *Cotton twin sets: one in navy, another in pink.*
15) *A white eyelet bustier worn under a white linen Spencer.*

In my notebook, I have recorded twenty additional ways she wore her skirt. In late September, when the days grew crisp and cool, she reached for her black cashmere turtleneck and belted it over the skirt. It's taken her years to collect all the components. She is a devoted markdown shopper and at least monthly trolls the outlet stores and a couple of her favorite addresses tucked away on obscure streets in neighborhoods I've only heard about to pick up finds for herself and her daughter.

In the winter, her wardrobe is centered upon lots of black. Red, though, is probably her favorite color, and she uses it to spike black. One of her favorites is a to-die-for long red redingote, which I gave to her, with a red velvet collar, cuffs, and frog closings. As you can see from the list above, my friend's predilection for Spencer jackets is absolute. She has one navy blazer, but only wears it with jeans. Sometimes she wears red jeans.

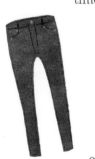

Chic vaguely translates as "stylish," but in my opinion that definition doesn't do the word justice. Chic does not come from an overflowing closet bursting with big name labels—that's easy. All a woman would need would be the wherewithal; chic has nothing to do with cash flow. Chic is an eclectic mix of high and low, new and old, scrambled together to reflect a woman's personality, i.e., her style. Why, a Frenchwoman asks, would she yearn to look like a hyper-tricked-out fashion magazine photograph, a brand's ad (read: head-to-

toe dumbed down coordination), or an actress who pays a stylist to dress her? Copying makes no sense to her way of thinking. "Where am *I* in the picture?" she asks herself.

Over tea in a Paris café, Marisa Berenson, who went from "It" girl to icon and along the way became a permanent fixture on the world's best-dressed lists, offered her particularly pertinent opinions on style. "What amazes me about certain women—we won't name names, let's just say non-Frenchwomen—is that they literally have their clothes worked out into 'outfits.' They have lists of what to wear, including how to accessorize. They don't want to make mistakes, I guess," she said. "I don't understand; maybe it makes their lives easier?"

I know of a woman who looks unfailingly well turned out in exceedingly expensive names from haute couture and ready-to-wear with all the accessories that one would expect— she doesn't "do" low, ever—but the effect is anything but "easy" or natural. She looks groomed to the point of sterility. The personality, the style spark is woefully missing, despite great effort and the labels. She has her maid photograph her before she leaves the house not only to confirm that her mission was accomplished, but also to ensure that in the future she will be certain to avoid the misstep of wearing the same ensemble with the same people.

(My friend Anne-Françoise applies the method above to dinner parties, where I see the logic. She has a large book in which she keeps the menus of her dinners, with a picture of the table and a list of the *invités*. As her guests, we anticipate with pleasure her creative table settings almost as much as her unfailingly delicious meals. In this case, she's thinking about us and our pleasure, and I can assure you we appreciate her efforts.)

Berenson, who says she never knows what she will wear from day to day and who doubts that she has "ever put anything together in the same way twice," and who certainly doesn't think of her clothes as preconceived outfits, knows how to accomplish her undertaking with *joie de vivre*. She enjoys the process and the fresh ideas that come to her as she regards the choices in front of her. Her closet inspires.

"Getting dressed is not a chore," she said. "When I have a big soirée, I do think in advance, but otherwise I open my closets and pull out things that are pleasing to me, that reflect my mood."

She cannot imagine angst associated with dressing.

I remarked to her that before I moved to France and even when I traveled back to the States for work, I often had the American mentality of believing it necessary to have a completely different outfit every day, ever avoiding the dreaded possibility of being seen several times in the same clothes, whereas Frenchwomen bask in the compliment "I love you in that dress." She laughed and said that was "so true. It's not about the new, the new. It's about feeling good in your clothes. That's when a woman has style."

STAYING NEUTRAL

Let's be clear: creating the perfect wardrobe takes time, discipline—yes, that word again—and a grand plan. Without those elements, chaos reigns. Chaos causes stress; stress causes wrinkles. Enough said.

One day, I saw a woman of indeterminate age—she could have been forty-five, she could have been sixty—wearing, from top to bottom, the following: an ecru, tissue-thin sweater T-shirt (I'm presuming cashmere); huge gold chain at the neck; nubby brown-tweed Spencer, nipped in at the waist; a straight, knee-length chocolate-brown leather skirt; dark brown opaque hose and mid-heel suede boots of the same color. Her just-above-the-shoulder blonde hair was just so without being too-too, and she was literally sprinting across the street to catch a taxi. Imagine the way those pieces would break out into possibilities.

I wanted to rip her clothes off of her and wear them home, except that she was probably a size six, max. Oh, and much shorter than I am.

Who can't wear some version of that look for the rest of her life? The effect would have been the same had the separates been an assemblage of other neutrals such as black, gray, or navy.

Frenchwomen of a certain age have built their wardrobes upon a foundation of neutrals. They add spice with a few magical, highly personal finds. That way they "own" the look. They are masters of the art-meets-science cocktail. Science is the structure. Art is the refinement, the individualization of the whole. It's the artistic twists that transform the ubiquitous into the unusual, the unique.

The woman I saw in the street, and at least 95 percent of the women I photograph on the street, no matter what the season, tend to be wearing neutrals of some sort. In the summer, it's whites and every imaginable nuance in the beige/greige/taupe family, navy blue, and the occasional little black dress in linen. In the winter, many tend to turn to black and gray in every hue from charcoal to putty. Others build upon the chocolate/*café au lait*/camel/toast family and, again, navy blue.

You've heard this before? Sometimes it's difficult to stay on message without frequent reminders, so here comes some repetition for emphasis if you will: Assuming every woman wants to have a fulfilling relationship with her clothes, one that defines her uniquely individual style, the elements must be supported by a solid foundation. A solid foundation is neutral. It's the reason why we need fewer bottoms—skirts and trousers, jeans—and many, many, many more tops. If a wardrobe features too many bottoms, it is fundamentally flawed. Is it really intelligent or efficient to have three gray-flannel knee-skimming pencil skirts; ten pairs of black pants; the same jeans, exact cut and color, five times over?

My friend Babette owns two boutiques in the town near our village—one is a shoe, belt, and bag shop, the other sells clothes. Babette knows what women want. Many of her most loyal clients are Parisians with country houses near us. Most of them work, she informed me. They love her taste—as my daughter and I do.

"I think what I do for women in my buying is to make their busy lives easier. They like the way I pull everything together. It's not that they couldn't find great things in Paris;

it simply takes more time. They know that they'll always find something *chez moi* that will add a new element to what they own."

She says 70 percent of the clothes in her boutique fall into neutral territory. "When I buy collections, inside each collection I buy 85 percent neutrals and 15 percent fantasy, as in color, cut, and/or details," she said.

"The women who shop here have strong personalities. They know what they like; they know what they need; they think before they buy," she added. "They have meetings, dinners, and some a country and a city life. They need clothes they can count on in many situations."

She showed me a traditional charcoal-gray wool blazer. The twist was the yellow or red patches on the elbows and the repeat of the color on the back of the turned-up collar. "A Frenchwoman of any age could wear that in a meeting or with a pair of jeans." Classic with a twist.

Her customers range in age from fourteen to eighty and many of them, regardless of age, are wearing the same pieces, assembled differently according to lifestyle.

Let's test the theory, I suggested.

I pulled a crepe ecru tunic—slight scoop neck, with a one-inch triangle print in Bordeaux, and full-ish long sleeves, gently gathered at the wrist and "push-up-able"—from a rack and asked her to "put this hypothetically on a mother and her daughter."

DAUGHTER: Charcoal leggings; high, solid, flat, black boots; cropped brown, leather jacket. The length could be adjusted with the self-tie belt of the tunic.

MOTHER: Bordeaux leggings; low, black, feminine *bottines* with a small heel; a narrow leather belt to adjust the waist to its most flattering position; "and a scarf to add a touch of elegance."

HOW THEY CONSTRUCT A *GARDE-ROBE*

For those of us who long to overhaul, and ultimately to streamline our wardrobes, here's the good news: it's not complicated. Time is required in the beginning, but once the foundation has been constructed, anxiety and doubt disappear.

This is the way Frenchwomen of a certain age have always done it:

THE GRAND PLAN: For novices, paper and pencil may be used. That's the way I did it. (I also keep a tiny Moleskin notebook in my bag at all times that has lists of what I already own. There's no need to tell you how many times I've bought the same black sweaters or white T-shirts.) The grand plan is based upon decisions that will lead us to clothes that are versatile and multifunctional.

THREE QUESTIONS MUST BE POSED AT THIS POINT:

1) Does everything I own flatter my figure?
2) Do the styles now represented in my wardrobe reflect my personality, the image I wish to project? If this question has never been posed, now's the time.
3) Does what I own fulfill my needs? Can I reach in

there and pull out something appropriate and pleasing for every moment of my life? That is what we call "dressing one's lifestyle."

Another consideration when assembling this marvelous creation known as "the perfect *garde-robe*": Frenchwomen fill their wardrobes with shapes and styles repeated over and over. They know which cuts fit and flatter. Any future experimentation is done in a boutique dressing room before a considered decision is made about the purchase of a new form of a jacket, or perhaps, instead of another pencil skirt, a pleated one might be fun for a change. They do this if, and only if, the latest items cohabit comfortably with pieces already hanging in their closets.

It's the details that make similar styles appear new.

Lagerfeld again: "Buy what you don't have yet, or what you really want, which can be mixed with what you already own. Buy only because something excites you, not just for the simple act of shopping."

One can literally find hundreds of different gray jackets, thousands of white blouses, scores of black skirts, and who-knows-how-many cuts of jeans.

Frenchwomen constantly build on and refresh their base color family. Don't think for a moment, "How boring." It's anything but. It's intelligent, ageless, and always, *always* chic. Best of all, it makes getting dressed so *easy*. Within the spectrum of neutrals, there are vast nuances of shades, textures, and possibilities.

Unexpected embellishments—buttons, embroidery,

piping, trims, surprising linings and insets, for example—can be built into a range of garments that are a consistent shape that works for a woman, but no one would know that the majority of her jackets are identical in cut. Frenchwomen raise the ante on the classic by seeking out items with unusual details.

ADDING COLOR

When I do my on-the-street photographs in Paris and in the country near our house (capturing two very contrasting types of dressing) for my blog, readers often ask me, "Where's the color?" Usually it's in the accessories; women of a certain age do succumb to color on occasion, but they show restraint in the dosages. Because Frenchwomen of a certain age have their basics covered, many have added color, usually along Babette's calculations of 15 to 20 percent.

Their color choices complement (and compliment) their neutrals; they are never one-offs. Orange in measured quantities goes with just about any color; therefore, an orange jacket or a skirt might be just what the season ordered. Klein blue is a French favorite and again poses no problems in a neutral wardrobe.

A flowered dress in the summer? Why not? But, I've noticed they're never large flowers, always along the scale of Liberty prints. How about Burgundy and all its wine companions? What can't be worn with a cabernet or Bordeaux? It's almost a neutral, though I think most women opening an armoire to discover a wine closet would find the hues depressing after the first heady encounters.

In my wanderings I have occasionally noticed one of the great exceptions to the neutral dictum: winter coats in primary, secondary, or pastel tones. Usually they are worn by women of a certain age who most certainly have had their basics well covered for years and want to add verve to their wardrobes in the gray months of winter.

But a wardrobe *based* upon color? Never.

Inevitably, basing a wardrobe on neutrals is the only way to produce major returns on investments.

Think about it: Bright colors and cacophonous prints? Nothing goes with anything. With neutrals, a woman can always pull something out of the closet and pull herself together without hysteria in record time. Everything goes together naturally. No mess, no stress.

A vibrant color and, on occasion, a single print item might rev up the base to acknowledge, "Yes, I'm *au courant* about what's going on this season." Frenchwomen are never slaves to fashion, but they're not oblivious to it either. They like an invigorating shot of the new and the now, but they never overdose on the ephemeral.

THREE QUESTIONS

First, ask yourself, is my house in order?
You must begin with wardrobe assessment, rejection, deconstruction, and reconstruction. No matter how many times we've heard this and in our heart of hearts know it's true, it's not necessarily easy. But it must be done. Harsh decisions must be made. Emotional attachments must be resolved.

At our age, we probably know what works best on our bodies. It's evident. It's those clothes we wear over and over, buy over and over, the items that receive the most compliments, not the ones hanging there unworn. If in doubt, it's never too late to find out. With the help of a mirror (preferably three-way), a friend who has a great—critical—eye, or perhaps an appointment with a personal shopper, a free service offered by major department stores, and a pile of clothes, uncertainty evaporates in no time at all.

It's a shame there isn't a-rent-a-French-friend service that could send over a chic *femme* to help whittle our closets into shape. Chances are she would be brutally honest in her assessment; Frenchwomen are "special" in that way.

Next on the agenda comes this question: Am I expressing my personality through my clothes?
Our clothes are our first unspoken message to the world. It seems only logical to use it. Why lose such a stunning opportunity? How we're turned out gives a lasting impression that according to some expert studies is transmitted in fewer than five seconds.

Finally, lifestyle plays a role in our closet construction projects. Do I own what I need and desire? Does my wardrobe function? Is it me?
If a woman's lifestyle is one where she works from home, either as a freelancer or raising her children, or she's no longer working and is inventing new adventures, she might think she doesn't need to "get dressed." *Non, non,*

non. It's *always* important for a woman to look her best. Frenchwomen never forget they are setting the standard for their partners, their children, and their grandchildren. They also know getting dressed is a major morale booster. I've had serious morale boosts myself from merely watching chic Parisians sauntering down the street.

FIT, FIT, FIT

Another detail I've noticed in my nearly microscopic scrutiny of the species is that my role models wear their clothes somewhat differently and slightly less tightly than they once did.

In their teens, twenties, and into their thirties, Frenchwomen are inclined to like their clothes cut *very* close to the body. As the decades roll on, everything loosens up a bit. Fabrics no longer snugly hug the figure, but instead gently embrace its curves. "Curves" is the operative word. "Feminine" is practically a synonym for Frenchwoman. When you see a Frenchwoman is wearing a pantsuit that at first seems masculine, look more closely and you'll note that the jacket is tailored to show the female form, and if the décolleté is holding up well or the *dermabrasion or mésothérapie* injections (please see skin chapter for my experience with the latter) worked, maybe there is nothing but a lacy bra or a froufrou bustier beneath the jacket.

One of the most masculine ensembles that exists is a man's tuxedo suit, but Yves Saint Laurent turned it into one of the sexiest, most feminine evening looks ever. The tuxedo, or "smoking," as the French call it, was redesigned to curve into and enhance feminine curves.

And while we're on the subject, most Frenchwomen of a certain age own a tuxedo (or two), maybe one in a dark midnight navy and another in black. They think of it as separates as well as a suit. You can see how that works. The jacket with black jeans, a white shirt or T-shirt, for example, the trousers with a black turtleneck . . . You get the picture.

RECASTING, EXPANDING, PLAYING

Frenchwomen like dresses, particularly in the summer. But unlike us, they do not pack them away the instant the calendar announces the arrival of autumn. Instead, they transition their dresses in the most charmingly inventive ways, while at the same time giving them a longer seasonal lifespan. They might put a turtleneck sweater over a sleeveless dress. Bare legs go undercover in opaque hose, and low heels or ballerinas usually replace sandals. Some more adventurous types break the rules and wear their tights with sandals. (It works for them. What can I say? It looks quirky, but never dowdy.) Classic long-sleeved sweaters or buttoned-up cardigans, often belted, turn the dresses into skirts. Jean jackets take the edge off the softness of summery *robes*. Scarves that may have been reluctantly stored on the shelf during the hotter months come flying out of their safe haven.

It was a gray day in early October when I ran in to visit Babette, and there she was in her version of summer-meets-fall. She was wearing a navy cotton shirtdress; navy opaque tights; tan one-inch chunky heeled lace-up *bottines;* and since it was slightly nippy, she'd slipped on a cropped beige

V-neck cardigan with a floppy red silk poppy "brooch," one of her autumn/winter buys for her boutique. (The poppy came with the sweater—details, details, details.) Her fingernails were the same color as the poppy.

HOW SOME OF THE WOMEN DO IT

Anyone who has seen or met Marisa Berenson would certainly agree that she, in her highly personal interpretation of style, is the ultimate barometer of all things chic and unique. She lives much of the time in Paris, and one tends to think of her as *being* French, although she is not.

Her father was an American career diplomat and her mother a countess with Italian, Swiss, French, and Egyptian ancestry. And, of course, her maternal grandmother was the surrealism-inspired designer Elsa Schiaparelli. Some might say she was born to be a star, and one of the world's most naturally elegant at that. She does reflect all the qualities one imagines as the French ideal: modulated voice, impeccable manners, feminine gestures, charm, and, most certainly, that original style.

Berenson likes color. We've seen her in the occasional neutral, but her style is more exuberant than the typical Frenchwoman's. Perhaps that comes from her Italian heritage and her mother's and grandmother's influence. Another woman who not only influenced Berenson, but also launched her fabulous fashion career, was the divine Diana Vreeland, the woman who, as editor, made *Vogue* vogue, and who later moved on to the Metropolitan Museum of Art, where she had yet another of her brilliant ideas:

glamorous costume exhibits launched by gala A-list soirées where what-are-they-wearing watching is unparalleled.

It was clear in our interview that examining the finer points of style comes as naturally to Berenson as getting dressed in the morning.

"I think Frenchwomen have a sense of self," she said. "They understand that dressing is personality. It seems to me that Americans are preoccupied with a certain kind of perfection; Frenchwomen are not. If you feel good about yourself, you don't need endless changes of clothes or unlimited cash. If you look good, you look good."

Berenson did admit that the essence of style is innate. "It's daring to put personality into dressing," she said.

She also said she suspects many women don't know themselves well, and thus their unique styles elude them. In a fashion magazine article, she mused about the possibility that true individuality may be evaporating.

"I think there are very few people who have a real style, a real personality, and real beauty. Everything sort of melts into everything else," she said.

She has a point, but I prefer to address her advice for finding one's style: know thyself.

Accepting the proposition that style is personality is the first giant step toward achieving it, I would think. All of the Frenchwomen I know well and those I met for the first time for this book express their vastly different personalities with their clothes and accessories.

Anne-Marie de Ganay, for example, is considered one of the most chic women in Paris. After spending an afternoon with her, which included a visit to her vast cavern of a closet, I understood not only why, but also how she earned her reputation.

Regrettably I can't even aspire to one aspect of her how-to tricks—she has an enviable collection of haute couture, which, as you know, often comes at prices comparable to the cost of an Ivy League college education. Never mind—her couture is snuggled right up against some of her great finds from Parisian street markets (you would be surprised at the wonders one can find a few steps from the vegetables) and Zara, which she proclaimed is one of her "favorite places to shop." She also likes Monoprix on occasion. We *all* love Monoprix, a smaller, more chic, more refined, extremely French Target, where you jump with joy when you realize you can afford everything on offer, including that great *marinière* (sailor T-shirt) in cashmere with brass buttons on the shoulder.

"Have I changed the way I've always dressed?" she asked rhetorically. "No, honestly I don't think I have. I wear different designers and get a *petit frisson* out of finding a little jacket at Zara, or a satin, pleat-front shell I found recently and wore under one of my embroidered jackets from India with a pair of large satin trousers to a black-tie event."

If a woman wears only one designer and never mixes it up, not only is she missing out on a good time, but also "she looks plastic," Ganay declared.

Her casual stay-at-home attire includes leggings, a large man's shirt, and ballerina flats. Often she'll add something from her extensive ethnic jewelry collection.

She also loves long skirts, which I consider difficult to pull off with panache. She does it, though.

Anne de Fayet was one of the first women I met when we moved to France. At the time she was the public relations director of the Comité Colbert, the prestigious organization of French luxury brands that promotes French *art de vivre*.

We became friends through our work relationship and have kept in touch on and off over the years. She incarnates my idea of the ultimate in French chic—a rich mélange of classic refinement that is so subtly sumptuous that she has always been one of my favorite role models. For as long as I've known her she has been a part of *la mode*, but never a fool for fashion. I remember one autumn, an American friend and I attended a cocktail party, convinced we were smartly and stylishly attired—after all, we had both lived in France long enough to know what to wear to a cocktail party, for heaven's sake—until in walked Anne de Fayet. No glitz, no la-di-da, simply pure refinement in a new dress that proclaimed the latest fall trend in exquisite understatement. Simple, sober, elegant: what more could one desire? Jean and I gave each other a withering she-just-did-it-again look and headed off for our second flutes of champagne.

Anne proved the possibility that being "on message" for the latest and the greatest from a current fashion cycle does not preclude long-term investment. That cocktail party was at least ten years ago, and I'm sure she continues to wear the dress.

On the day we met for a glass of wine to talk about style, elegance, and charm, Anne was wearing a charcoal flannel pencil skirt; a lighter gray long-sleeve cashmere T-shirt cinched with a one-inch brown belt; a light-brown collarless leather jacket; black opaque tights; black ballerina flats; and gum-ball-sized gray pearls that I assumed to be real.

One of the turns in our conversation was how Anne responded to questions on style. She chose to address, not the dress, but rather the woman within. "Trying too hard conveys a message of insecurity," she said. "Elegance comes through in so many elements that it can never be attributed solely to what a woman wears. Clothes do not make a woman elegant; it's the woman who makes the clothes elegant. It's the way she moves, speaks, applies her makeup with a light hand, has a great haircut and just the right color; it's a combination of details."

Eh, oui, the devil is *always* in the details.

As Yves Saint Laurent said: "Over the years I have learned that what is important in a dress is the woman who is wearing it."

I asked a few of the women I interviewed to describe their perfect start-from-scratch wardrobes. In other words, if I were to swoop into their closets and remove everything they owned and they had to buy the basics, what would they choose? This is what Anne told me:

1) Two skirts, "probably straight," one gray, one black.

2) A well-tailored pantsuit in espresso.

3) A moss-green velvet jacket.

4) Gray trousers.

5) A black cashmere twin set.

6) Classic cashmere pullovers in gray and black, plus turtlenecks in the same colors.

7) A brown leather jacket.

8) Levi's jeans.

9) An ecru satin blouse.

10) Two large cotton chemises, cut like men's shirts.

11) My ten-year-old little black dress.

"I don't like color, therefore there isn't a lot of it in my wardrobe," she admitted. Like her contemporaries, she shops at Zara, as well as Mango on occasion. We all seem to agree that a cashmere T-shirt from Monoprix is a good short-term investment. It's also a reasonably priced way to buy a season's "in" color without breaking the bank.

I've known Genevieve Guerlain for almost as long as I've lived in France. We met at a dinner party at a mutual friend's house not long after Andrea and I settled into our tiny village. Genevieve and her family have a country house not far from us. She is stunning. Like Anne de Fayet, who is a good friend of hers, she dresses with utter simplicity, but it's not the *same* simplicity. Her style is microscopically less nonchalant. It's slightly crisper, less *décontracté* (relaxed).

She invited me to lunch at her apartment in Paris to discuss her take on style. On the day we met, Genevieve was wearing a short-sleeved pale toast-colored wool crepe shift that gently skimmed her body. A large brooch perched majestically high to the right of the dress's simple round neck, and on her feet were brown suede Roger Vivier heels.

When I put her to the wardrobe test, this is what she told me:

1) Two tailleurs (suits), each with a skirt and a pair of trousers.

2) Two little black dresses, one like the dress I'm wearing today and another one.

*3) A collection of cashmere sweaters: two black with long
sleeves, one turtleneck, one round neck, one gray, one
brown, one moss green.*

4) A classic, well-cut blazer.

"I love wearing my old clothes," she said. "They make me
feel comfortable and I'm sentimental about some of them."

She added, "At the moment I'm tired of trousers, so
for the last six months I've been wearing dresses most of
the time."

HOW TO DRESS LIKE A *FEMME FRANÇAISE D'UN CERTAIN ÂGE*: THE PROS EXPLAIN

My first job after graduating from college was with
Women's Wear Daily, which many consider the
graduate school of fashion journalism. One of our
regular assignments, after the ready-to-wear collections,
whether we worked out of New York or any of the bureaus
across the United States and Europe, was to interview
the women (and sometimes the men) who bought the
clothes they saw on the runways.

The drill was to ask them specifically what they ordered.

These were the individuals who saw beyond the
theatrics in the shows, had front-row views of all the collections one after the other (total immersion), and had close
relationships with the designers. They were the ones who
mixed it all up, mingling their vision of style with *la mode*
of the moment. They instinctively saw the possibilities and

bought accordingly, whether they were the fashion directors of large stores or owned their signature boutiques.

Today, Maria Luisa Poumaillou is considered one of the grand masters of the art. Journalists turn to her to pose questions about the latest and the greatest, while faithful clients rely on her counsel to help them integrate her finds into their wardrobes.

She and her husband, Daniel, opened their first boutique, the eponymous Maria Luisa, in 1988. In record time, her reputation as a fashion star in a galaxy dominated by individual designers was recognized internationally. With her strong point of view and discerning eye for the new and the next, she created a boutique with great style and personality. She recently closed the shop to concentrate on an ever-evolving in-house boutique on the second floor of the famous Paris department store Printemps, whose flagship is housed in a beautiful belle-époque building.

It's an ideal partnership for the woman who is credited with putting such names as Martin Margiela, Ann Demeulemeester, Helmut Lang, Rick Owens, Alexander McQueen, Nicolas Ghesquière, Christopher Kane, and others on the fashion radar.

On the late spring day when we met in her offices near the rue de Rivoli, she was wearing black silk trousers ("three years old"); a large, black silk boat-neck dolman sleeve blouse of her own design ("one year old"); and a white linen blazer ("six years old"), cuffs turned back, again cut on the large side. She had a big, black-resin cuff bracelet on one wrist; a wide black belt ("eight years old"); a large, flat pearly gray shell that hung around her neck on a black leather cord and almost touched the belt's buckle; hoop earrings; black low-heeled *bottines;* black sunglasses; and red, red lipstick.

You see, classic but not. She had the components of an ensemble that could have been uptight, boring, or disturbingly buttoned-up. Instead, the effect was slouchy chic. It was the cut of the clothes that made the difference.

What I love about Poumaillou is that she's on our side. She says she wants the clothes she buys to flatter, not merely to mark a fashion moment or glorify a designer.

"Let's face it, if a woman isn't comfortable in her clothes, she can never be stylish," she said. "Take the blazer-pencil skirt look for example. I find it 'hard.' I prefer 'soft.'" That being said, her "soft" is never froufrou; she has a way of finding clothes that round the edges off the tough.

She thinks we should be wearing more skirts, but unlike many designers and fashionable women, she thinks we should consider full skirts, "particularly if a woman has pretty legs." She drew a picture of her ideal skirt for me, pointing out how it marks the waist. What she drew was not an A-line skirt, which she finds *dadame* (matronly). She prefers hemlines to hit one inch above the knee. "Under the knee is aging," she maintained.

When I asked her what she would have in her hypothetical wardrobe, she told me the following:

1) *Light cashmere sweaters: V-neck and ballet-neck in black, ecru, emerald, red, and khaki.*

2) *T-shirts, including a collection of debareurs, i.e., with a sleeveless, round neck.*

3) *Blue jeans, but never, never* delavé *(stone-washed):*
   "They're banal and should be left for the girls. We should be wearing dark blue jeans."

4) *Poplin shirts, including one in black and one in pale blue, as well as white, of course.*

5) *A perfectly cut blazer, one in black, one in navy. Depending upon budget considerations, she recommended Balenciaga, Joseph, and Theory. (Don't forget, if those price points are out of the question, a lesson can be learned from observation, markdown miracles sometimes happen, and remember, men's blazers are usually better made than many women's blazers and are considerably less expensive. They can be tailored to flatter a woman.)*

6) *A soft leather Spencer jacket.*

7) *Simple round-neck sweaters in vibrant colors.*

8) *Crepe de chine shirts in ecru and black.*

9) *A trench coat: "I have one in a panther print I've worn for years."*

10) *A long skirt. "They're always useful and can be dressed up or down. I have a long georgette skirt in a print I particularly like."*

Poumaillou believes that we should succumb to a *coup de foudre* (literally "struck by a thunderbolt," but commonly and figuratively an emotional love-at-first-sight reaction to someone or something) when shopping.

She has nothing against ethnic style if one is drawn to it, but she cautions against being preoccupied by *les tendances*. "Always find something for you, something that expresses who you are," she said. "Start with your morphology and work from there." She is an anti–status symbol advocate and believes designer labels should be left to the insecure and those who have money to waste.

And finally, perhaps the best piece of advice she offered was the simplest: "Never go against your instincts." Most of us have at one time, and we know those are the decisions that remain unworn in the back of the closet.

A DAY WITH A PERSONAL SHOPPER

Writing this book gave me the impetus to explore an opportunity I've always dreamed about pursuing: visiting a personal shopper, and a French one at that.

I called up the public relations department of Galeries Lafayette, the other famous Paris department store, and asked if someone could please assist me in my quest. Immediately—and I can assure you that "immediately" is not necessarily a concept employed by public relations people in France—a meeting was set up with Pascale. We spoke twice on the phone before our meeting. She wanted to know 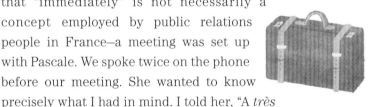 precisely what I had in mind. I told her, "A *très* Parisian wardrobe for women ranging in age from forty-ish to forever-ish." I also mentioned that this capsule collection should be kind to a variety of body types while maintaining the French touch.

Let me say upfront, I recommend a visit to Galeries Lafayette's personal shopping offices. When I arrived,

Pascale had set up a collection of pre-dressed mannequins, plus several changes of clothes for each; racks of little black dresses, separates, coats, jackets, and tops for me to peruse; plus shelves of accessories and covetable shoes marching around the perimeter of the huge apartment-like space on the top floor of the store. The view from the top is spectacular. All I could think was, I would like to move right in. Imagine the lifestyle. The kitchen was fully equipped to serve busy women who need their strength to keep on shopping, shopping, shopping, and all the clothes they could ever need would be a short elevator ride away. Never mind—I was there to work.

Before we examined her ensembles, I asked Pascale about style, which theoretically she is crafting for her clients. "Style, is 'allure' above all else," she said. "It's the way a woman walks, her gestures, her personality."

Inevitably, we return again to the idea that it's the woman who wears the clothes and not the reverse.

I think Pascale showed genius in assembling our "what if/only if" ageless *garde-robe*. I say "only if" because most of her choices were big-ticket items, but that is not important. It's the look, the shape, and the ideas that count.

Karl Lagerfeld agrees, which is reassuring. He's been quoted as saying, "Never use the word 'cheap.' Today everybody can look chic in inexpensive clothes (the rich buy them, too). There is good clothing design on every level today. You can be the chicest thing in the world in a T-shirt and jeans—it's up to you." So *voilà*.

Pascale had tricks for everything from unexpected

combinations of separates—think silver-sequined blazer with white jeans—to streamlined slimming ploys.

To look slim and chic, she kept the elements clean and classic. She teamed a straight black-leather skirt with a thinly knit, long-sleeved black scoop-neck sweater topped with a three-quarter trench coat featuring a leopard lining, sleeves turned back to reveal the motif. Her addition of a huge, two-strand chunky necklace in fat, translucent amber-colored beads sent the eyes right up to the face, where she had turned up the collar of the coat.

She then took the trench coat, which as we know goes with everything, including a cocktail or evening dresses, to another register by putting it with black cotton pants and a black-and-white-striped sailor sweater, leopard in evidence. Details.

She put a once-in-a-lifetime—but you need good arms—white cotton eyelet dress on one of the mannequins she had dressed for the occasion. The shape was perfection, beginning with a sleeveless top skimming down into a gentle, as in not clingy, empire waist, moving along flatteringly flat until the top of the thighs, where the skirt spun out. A jean jacket or a cardigan would solve the pesky arm problem.

Like many Frenchwomen, Pascale really, really likes white jeans and trousers, which she proved go with just about anything including, in one example, a black-sequined blazer with a black-and-white-striped T-shirt beneath.

Another of her ageless combinations: a deep, deep V-neck cashmere sweater in ecru, tucked into a pleated tan skirt, belted. Not complicated. Very pretty, very pure. Zero accessories. Elegant.

We were having nonstop fun, and, of course, by this point I was dreaming about having a trust fund. Moving right along, she next added a creamy soft, black zip-front cardigan-like leather jacket to the tan skirt and ecru sweater and a clever scarf trick to change the entire mood.

She paired an absolutely classic pair of black cotton trousers with a black-and-white seersucker blazer and a white, long-sleeved V-neck T-shirt. The look was fresh and young.

She proved, if any of us need convincing—and I definitely did—that a jean jacket is a necessity. She showed it two ways, both with dresses: one a black-and-white V-neck T-shirt piped in red at the neck and hem with a red inset "belt"; the other option a small, ladylike silk print in muted blues, white, and coral. She used a straightforward brown leather menswearlike belt to meld the contrasting tough and tender.

As I said, Frenchwomen like their white trousers. She redressed a mannequin, this time with a bright, bright orange silk blouse featuring deep cowl folds. Think Vanessa Bruno.

We all love the ring of the word "investment" when used in the same sentence with "clothes." I asked her what she thought would be one of those ultimate wear-for-the-rest-of-one's-life purchases. "A deep, midnight-blue tuxedo," she said. Who doesn't rhapsodize about *le smoking* in its purest form, nothing beneath the jacket, just the woman, and then dream about the myriad possibilities of the jacket with almost any skirt or trousers? The trousers on their own with a cashmere sweater, a white men's shirt. The jacket with jeans, sublime.

Pascale decreed that one could, probably should, own a blazer or two and then produced one shimmering with silver sequins, another in black sequins. *Oh-là-là*. A woman would never need another idea for what to wear to a party. Either would be swoon-worthy with the tuxedo pants. She proved the silver looked like it belonged with a pair of white trousers.

And, finally, Pascale, where should a woman put her money? "In a coat," she said without hesitation. (Maria Luisa Poumaillou agreed.)

Toward the end of our day together, Pascale led me over to a long rack where she had assembled a collection of every imaginable nuance on the little black dress.

My favorite, and I didn't bother glancing at the price, was a silk crepe Azzedine Alaïa: round neck, V at the back, three-quarter sleeves, and pleats sewn down from beneath the bust to the thighs, constructed in such a way that the seams whittled the waist and caressed the hips, almost like a corset but without the constraint, then came the liquid pleats, which moved in the most seductive way. Even on a hanger, one could imagine how they would float around a woman's legs. I could envision the way a woman would feel wearing that dress—fatally feminine, powerfully alluring. That, in a nutshell, is what the French understand about clothing: that it has the power to transform us, to entertain us, to change our self-images, and occasionally even to change our lives.

The Essential
Accessory Arsenal

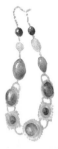

EVERY WOMAN'S NECESSARY
ACCOUTREMENTS

Accessories are fascinating. They deliver the power, the personality, the panache that can quietly or boldly communicate a woman's confidence and creativity. Accessories say more about personal style than the clothes they enhance. It's not difficult to construct a chic, workable wardrobe once a woman finds the basics that work for her, but it's the addition of singularly individual accoutrements that add her indelible, personal flair.

And this is where Frenchwomen of a certain age excel. In this domain, one must be acutely alert to appropriate their sleight of hand. They're very clever. It's Frenchwomen's creative, sometimes flamboyant, eminently personal use of accessories that sets them apart and makes everything old look new again. Or, which I find infinitely more intriguing, that makes *la mode* irrelevant.

Accessories perform the tricks that allow a French-woman to wear the same little black dress for twenty-five years. (That, of course, coupled with her calorie intake and perhaps a good seamstress when, despite all her mighty efforts, she may still need to add sleeves to a beloved sleeveless classic or release the waist a smidge.)

To be perfectly honest, I've reached the point where I'm ready to call a sleeve an accessory, and my extraordinary seamstress, Madame Sneady, knows how to add sleeves seamlessly, as in no one knows but the two of us. One would think the garment was originally designed with arm cover. She's also capable of turning 1980s shoulders on outrageously expensive jackets and coats into snug, snappy *au courant* styles. To remain on subject, I'm calling shoulder pads accessories. In a sense they are.

Those are the famous under-the-radar tweaks for which Frenchwomen of a certain age are so famous. Clothes are the canvas. Accessories are where the artistry comes in, transforming the simplest garment into a head-turning stunner, while at the same time eloquently proclaiming the taste and personality of the woman wearing them.

After years of covering fashion collections throughout the world, it was obvious to me that accessories are usually the key element in making a designer's work, well, work. By observing both sides—the runway and the women in the audience—I learned my most lasting lessons. If I ever had a doubt, that it's *always* all about the details, it was dispelled.

Still, for many years, I was a timid accessorizer—a bright bag; a few slim, gold bangles my mother had given me birthday by birthday over the years; a single strand of pearls (never a fabulous look-at-me mass à la Chanel); a scarf (never a shawl, they kept falling off); red or bright violet-blue leather gloves. The problem was that I was not making a statement. There was no coherence, no vision. I wasn't expressing my personality. I was simply throwing on an embellishment without thinking about impact. I wasn't applying my French lessons. And, to be perfectly honest, I was missing out on a lot of fun.

Those days are long over. And fortunately, if curiously perhaps, I always *bought* plenty of accessories, even when I was wearing them parsimoniously. They were right there in my closet: scarves and shawls heaped on several shelves; more shoes than we need to mention; a few great bags; belts, belts, belts; gloves; tons of pearls; a lovely jewelry box filled with a nice collection of real and semiprecious pieces begging to be mixed together and worn with panache; even a few hats.

Now I cannot live without my accessories, even when I'm sitting in front of my computer. A scarf has become a piece of clothing for me—I feel as if something is "off" if I'm not wearing one.

Every day, even when I leave the house only to buy a baguette, I wear the following: large-ish gold *créole* earrings (hoop earrings, a French classic); a scarf—winter, spring, and fall—my mother's collection of five, slender gold bangles with my men's Cartier tank watch (same wrist—

quelle élan!); ballerina flats or moccasins—sometimes in amusing colors or leopard print, paired in the winter with brightly colored socks; and my can't-live-without dark tortoise Ray-Ban Wayfarer sunglasses (I'm mad about them). They're also prescription and thus allow me to drive to the *boulangerie* without hitting a tree.

These days, when I wear pearls, I *wear* pearls. Not only that, but I have multiple strands in pink and gray, as well as in white. The pink are surprisingly pretty mixed with my coral necklaces, the gray with a string of chunky peridot beads. The turquoise necklaces I collected while living in Albuquerque, New Mexico, and my favorites given to me by my beloved mother-in-law are so much more sophisticated now when I wear them with my lapis beads. Blue on blue, so chic. I'm convinced I've learned—okay, let's say "absorbed"— these rather unexpected combinations by watching the inventiveness Frenchwomen bring to accessorizing.

Coco Chanel liberated women twice, first from their corsets and then by proving it was unspeakably chic to wear faux jewels. She also liked to mix them up with the real thing. Frenchwomen are always redefining the possibilities.

Essentially, that's the sole *raison d'être* for accessories: to mix it up, make the most out of the least, to show individuality and personality through the elements we can so easily control. And they're *so* much fun.

We can collect like a curator. On a clothes-buying expedition, we're often searching for something to wear for a specific reason, a special occasion, but that is rarely the case when shopping for accessories. We can take our time, fall in love, accumulate with acuity.

My favorite French fashion magazines are the spring and fall issues that proclaim in bold type, *ACCESSOIRES!* They help us sift through the news and see how some of the accessories were worn in the collections and then reimagined by the stylists for the magazine.

Frenchwomen, like many of us, use their magazines for news and reference. The desire for information is primordial for all of us. However, one major difference prevails between their magazines and ours: nowhere will you find how-to's or lists of do's and don'ts in theirs.

Call it subtle, call it subversive, but the message is clear: Frenchwomen can think for themselves, pick up the clues subliminally, and act on the information they've accumulated by perusing the pages filled with fashion news. They don't need directions. I see the accessory issues, as do my girlfriends, they tell me, as the "actionable" issues. Before we decide whether we really *need* more clothes, we know we definitely *want* more accessories. These, too, are the issues that offer the most ideas about how to wear the details that make all the difference. The news is obvious from the photos, no wordy explanations are necessary—or offered.

Luckily, accessories are the arena where fashion declarations can be made without breaking the bank—a leopard-print purse, zebra ballerinas, a lime-green snake-skin belt, a silver tote, masses of colored beads, whatever. Accessories were created to do what the dictionary describes as adding "an optional part that may be fitted to something to enhance performance."

Precisely. Literal translation: those special objects that enhance and extend the options of what's already hanging in our closets.

Accessories are always an easy first step into a new season. Let me explain: the vast majority of Frenchwomen of a certain age live primarily in neutrals—black, gray, navy, or the beige/brown/camel families. No matter. It's the addition of a scarf, a shawl, a shoe, a belt, a cuff bracelet, a pair of gloves, a necklace perhaps, or a combination of the above, that announces instantly, "I'm on message."

When silver bags were "in" for a nanosecond, my pal Françoise, who wears only Marithé et François Girbaud (which already tells you everything about her style), opted for a big one in polyurethane instead of leather, thus audaciously announcing that she was aware of what was going on but had no intention of spending major euros on the fad.

Brigitte, an acquaintance who owns an antique shop in the town near ours, wears only silver jewelry and lots of it. She piles on the same pieces every day with everything. It's her signature.

"One thing, though—I never wear earrings," she said. "They're not me. I can't explain it. I have wanted to wear *créoles* for years, but I'm not comfortable in them. The jewelry I wear every day is 'me.' I feel naked without it."

Her everyday assemblage includes: an armload of bangles in various widths and designs, rings, and one or several necklaces. Sometimes she wears a single amulet on a black silk cord; at other moments she may add more charms and more chains.

Another acquaintance, Nadege de Noilly, and I had lunch recently. She was decked out in jeans; a white T-shirt that exposed her collarbone; a long, filmy pale coral-and-ecru Jean Paul Gaultier blouse/dress/coat (very pretty); and *la pièce de résistance*: around her neck, she wore a wire she had made by her jeweler, dripping big charms, some with gems, some with engraved messages, some inherited, and others given to her over the years by her husband and children.

"It is so much a part of me, I keep touching it all day long," she said. "It is so simple, really. I asked my jeweler to make an eighteen-karat 'wire' strong enough to hold what would become the equivalent of a charm bracelet, but I prefer my charms to be around my neck. I wear it all the time with everything."

It's to-die-for gorgeous and, as she pointed out, when her husband or children cannot think of a gift, they give her one more charm. Each one is slightly larger than a quarter, each one preciously personal.

Now, let's get down to the specifics.

Since intelligent organization is a major part of a fashionable Frenchwoman's life, I thought I would apply orderliness to accessories, examining not only the necessary basics, but also the accoutrements that allow us to make personal statements without uttering a word. Very French indeed.

CHAPEAUX (HATS)

Regrettably, except for warmth, weddings, and warding off the sun, women have few hats in their closets.

Sweet knit cloches and berets appear on the streets when the temperatures dip, and French weddings always feature amazing hats, as do some of the more chichi horse races, most particularly the Prix de Diane in Chantilly, where there is major competition for the most unusual— which sometimes means bizarre—creations. We love these hats and the women who dare to wear them.

The house of Dior and a couple of other designers have tried to convince women they wanted to wear *capelines*, enormous hats that can touch the shoulders. The only way to describe them is as huge picture hats that look like they've melted.

Recently, Panama hats were everywhere—not only in natural hues, but also in every imaginable color. It was a fleeting moment, but oh-so-lovely.

SACS (BAGS)

A Frenchwoman's bag and shoes never match—yours don't either, I assume, even if they're in the same color family. She might choose patent leather for her shoes, suede for her bag. Texture changes everything.

As for purses, some prefer one Kelly, Birkin, or Chanel 2.55 in a major knockout color, a singular means of making an individual statement. With a little luck (and perseverance)

a snappy hue can sometimes be found in a Parisian secondhand designer apparel and accessory boutique. Others, often those who are convinced they will only own one major investment bag in their lifetimes, opt for the safe choices of black or brown.

There is an absolutely stunning woman in Paris who allows me to photograph her for my on-the-street blog feature. I've photographed her several times, but I've never asked her name. Except for summer, when she prefers a straw bag, she has a Birkin slung over her arm. However, it's never the *same* Birkin. She has a wardrobe of them: brown, lime, mauve, red—maybe more, who knows? Her other omnipresent accessory is a feisty Jack Russell.

It would be untrue if I told you I see nothing but designer bags on the street or among my friends. I've found that a Frenchwoman of a certain age much prefers to find a *sac* that will be different from anything else one might see. Frenchwomen go to great lengths to seek out obscure designers and boutiques that offer only the unusual, and there they find their special it's-all-about-me bags.

Maria Luisa Poumaillou, considered one of the fashion world's leaders for her remarkable talent in finding new designers and filling her boutiques—past and present—with clothes and accessories culled with the eye of an artist, is appalled by accoutrements that are, by definition, obvious status symbols.

"I don't understand how anyone wishes to say, 'I belong to a certain group of people,' through an accessory," she said. "I hate anything that screams 'brand.'"

We've often heard that necessity is the mother of invention. Vanessa Bruno told me that being a mother led her to invent perhaps her most well-known accessory.

The eye-catching design for her now famous and much copied canvas tote with sequin-splashed handles was a solution to a very personal need. "When my daughter was born I was carrying around so many things—the usual items a woman carries in her bag, as well as what I was working on at the time, and then the things a baby needs, including her bottle," she explained.

She simply wanted a bag that would be pretty as well as useful.

Pascale, the delightful personal shopper from Galeries Lafayette who spent hours talking with me about style and substance, is another advocate of finding the unusual when it comes to that oh-so-personal purse purchase. She proffered designer options, of course, but quickly pointed out that unusual, well-made, reasonably priced alternatives abound.

CHAUSSURES (SHOES)

As for shoes, it's not simply a question of "If the shoe fits . . . "
A *femme d'un certain âge,* like the rest of us, will not wear shoes in which she can't walk properly. Heel heights are chosen accordingly.

"Do I wear towering heels?" Chantal Thomass, the designer of super-saucy underpinnings, who has a reputation to maintain, mused rhetorically. "I certainly do, but not in the way I once did. I wear comfortable shoes in the car and slip on the stilettos right before my foot hits the pavement as I walk into a party."

Those who, like Chantal Thomass, save their sky-high heels for special occasions—read: moments of limited time and movement—never forget that ballerinas and moccasins are chic, ageless, and speed friendly. I see women in their seventies and beyond who understand a ballerina flat is always a better alternative to "sensible shoes"—or, more to the point they *are* their sensible shoes. Frenchwomen of a certain age prove every day that elegance and comfort are not mutually exclusive.

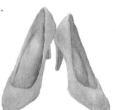

Frenchwomen of every age have collections of ballerinas and at least a couple of pairs of moccasins in their closets. Each is also booted up with a pair or two of high, soft leather boots—one in black, one in brown, one with a heel, one without. In most cases, a Frenchwoman probably also owns one pair of flat and another pair of mid-heel *bottines*, which are teamed with pants or opaque hose and a skirt. Worn in those ways, contrary to conventional wisdom, ankle-grazing boots have no age limit.

Even if she's wild about shoes and has an embarrassingly large collection (I believe some of us can identify with this particular obsession), she will always have the basics well covered: black kid, suede, and patent-leather pumps, slingbacks for spring and summer, nude leather for whenever. Depending upon her neutral wardrobe foundation, her shoes, bags, and belts will either add more dimension to that spectrum or add frank, bold punctuations of color.

Forthright hues such as ruby, sapphire, emerald, fuchsia, strong mauves, lime green, coral, and cobalt add effective embellishment. For evening, she has a pair of strappy sandals, black satin pumps, and ballerinas—at least one in a deep jewel tone. She probably has gold or bronze sandals, particularly flattering with a tan or naturally dark skin tones. She loves her espadrilles, flat or wedged, in the summer, and by this stage in her life, probably owns several pairs of flat sandals for warm weather months.

As I've mentioned throughout, French-women are frugal, and they rely on a handful of "enablers," those men and women who allow them to keep their clothes and accessories in pristine condition, sometimes for decades.

Monsieur Cotte is one of my enablers. He is my shoe man, but he is so much more. He has saved shoes I thought were lost forever, sewn sandals back together, and re-soled (and re-soled) some of my favorite shoes, and on the fun side, he has dyed several pairs multiple times. I had a pair of yellow slingback ballerinas. When it became clear the yellow was beyond salvation, he dyed them fuchsia; when fuchsia was so over, we moved on to Bordeaux. I figure they can one day be navy and, finally, black. He dyed my camel suede ballerinas bottle-green. We're now on a regular repair schedule: boots in at the end of the season for heel and sole check, maybe a polish. All shoes brought back to new immediately. He's a wizard.

Now is as good a time as ever to get the issue on and off the table. What about sport shoes? Yes, what about them? Doesn't the use of the noun "sport" as an adjective tell us something? Designed for sports. Yes, I'm not deaf to the argument about comfort and support, particularly when traveling, I'm told, but honestly, can't we do better than that? What ruins everything more efficiently and effectively than a pair of "sport shoes"?

Derbies, which can be wildly amusing, offer support. Well-constructed moccasins do the same. Converse high-tops are seen as often on Frenchwomen of a certain age as their daughters and granddaughters. Frenchwomen are also drawn to feminine sneakers, the most coveted brand being Bensimon. They're much like the classic Keds Americans wore to camp and which have, I've noticed, evolved enormously fashion-wise since those days.

BIJOUX, BIJOUX, BIJOUX (JEWELRY)

Ah, my favorite category.

Jewels, except for whimsical *bijoux de fantasie*, are the most personal of accessories, because they so often include heirlooms and sentimental memory markers. These are the pieces that can be so much an extension of a woman that they become part of her personality.

In France, they include pearls, of course, received as a sixteenth birthday present; charm bracelets, maybe given at a younger age (it does take a while to fill them up); gold bangles of varying widths; and whatever rings have come into a woman's possession over the years. Other staples bought or given include *créoles* or hoop earrings of various dimensions in gold and silver, gold chains, and, if you are lucky, simple diamond earrings that generous ancestors or appreciative lovers may have bequeathed.

Berna Heubner, an American friend of mine who has lived in Paris more than thirty years, introduced me to Nadege of the extraordinary charm necklace. She calls Nadege her muse. When she saw the necklace, she swooned, ran out, and had it copied. She has been collecting big charms ever since. Nadege gave her the name of her jeweler; she also gave it to me. It seems to me Frenchwomen get a bad rap about not sharing their secrets. Everyone I know does.

A personal jeweler is the ultimate luxury, not for the reason you might think. He (or she) is the ultimate luxury because he can transform existing horrors into great beauties, saving you money in the process.

Pierre, my personal jeweler, converted a pretty diamond and sapphire ring from an old boyfriend into a lovely clasp on a nice string of opera-length pearls—a gift from my ex-husband—which I gave to my daughter as an engagement present.

Certainly scale is important in principle, but when it comes to jewelry, I see delicately petite women with major chunky bracelets, huge rings, big-link necklaces, massive brooches—and somehow it always works. Just to be on the safe side, I'll state the obvious: they're not wearing everything at the same time (usually). That's the thing about style: easy to recognize, difficult to classify. Though most definitely possible to learn.

Remember, a mirror is a woman's best friend. When too much truly is too much, remove the excess.

Anne-Marie de Ganay, an exceedingly chic acquaintance, collects ethnic jewelry from no specific country; her only criteria are big and colorful. Since her real family jewels meet the same criteria, everything mixes nicely together. "These pieces are so festive and gay," she said, beaming, as she reached for a box full of her treasures. "I can add these to a long skirt, a top from Zara, and off I go. What could be more chic?"

My best and oldest friend, Anne-Françoise, lived in Brazil for years and as a consequence has one of the most extraordinary self-collected and created collections of jewelry I have ever seen. She loves big, pastel semi-precious stones set off with diamonds. She has nothing against emeralds and rubies either.

Now that she's moved back to France, every time I see her rings and earrings, I wish I'd visited her in Rio. She also has an impressive collection of family *bijoux*. In the case of Anne-Françoise, I don't think I've ever seen her wear costume jewelry. She has the whimsy element covered with the real deal.

Whenever I see her, I examine her jewels and often remark that she is wearing something I haven't seen before. "Don't be silly," she says, "of course you have, I've had [this/

these] for years." (Though occasionally she'll say, "Oh, no, you haven't. Danny gave it to me for my birthday.")

Anne-Françoise has three daughters, one of whom is my daughter's first and best French friend, and all have been outfitted with extensive bijoux wardrobes, some trickling down from the family vaults, others gifts from their mother, made in Brazil.

I've noticed that Frenchwomen of a certain age have specific predilections when it comes to their jewelry. Not one seems to feel equally strongly about everything. Anne-Françoise is mad about rings, and she also likes brooches and earrings. She rarely wears necklaces except for a major stone strung on a gold chain. Anne-Marie piles on rings and bracelets. Catie wears a single big, fat white pearl threaded on a delicate gold chain all the time with everything, even when swimming. Marianne, from what I have seen, dabbles in many categories, but always wears her wide, as in half-inch, diamond-encrusted wedding band.

One close friend always wears a deep blue, round-cut sapphire ring surrounded by diamonds. A lucky girl might have received it as her engagement ring.

This bauble is anything but. It was given to my friend by her husband after more than twenty-five years of marriage when he decided he wanted to call the whole thing off. These types of gifts are referred to as *les cadeaux de rupture*—translation unnecessary, I assume.

The tradition dictates that when a serious relationship comes to an end, the man gives the woman an *adieu* gift. These mementos can be anything from a piece of jewelry of little or significant value to something as simple as a tiny bouquet of violets.

As it turned out, my friend's marriage did not end and she has become quite attached to the ring—upon seeing it, one understands immediately why.

I love earrings, really like bracelets, and have many, many necklaces I rarely wear, even though I've collected them with a passion over the years.

Watches. A Frenchwoman will usually have a single precious version she will wear most of the time and an "amusing" one that tends to come out in the summer. Some of my friends eschew fun altogether and wear their owned-forever-lots-of-memories classics every day.

I have two watches. One is a man's Cartier tank that gets occasional band changes, sometimes in bright colors. My husband gave me the other—a delicate diamond evening number on a black satin ribbon that belonged to his mother.

CEINTURES (BELTS)

Frenchwomen truly do make age irrelevant. Why would they stop wearing belts simply because they're not as wasp-waisted as they once were? If a detail poses a problem, they will rethink the challenge and find a solution. They much prefer that approach to giving in or giving up.

To accommodate their slightly thickening waistlines at this point in their lives, Frenchwomen of a certain age wear their belts differently: looser, lower, and over a layer instead of the old way of cinching them around their middles or threading them tightly through belt loops. Some find scarves are more forgiving in place of belts, especially with trousers.

Many like grosgrain ribbons, which are gentle, feminine, and can add a hint of a season's new color.

ÉCHARPES, FOULARDS, CHÂLES (SCARVES)

No question about it. This is where Frenchwomen are most in their element.

Prior to becoming a fashion journalist, I recall noticing scarves being worn in one of two ways: long, bulky knitted scarves wrapped around necks to keep them warm (I was born in Niagara Falls), and silk squares triangled and tied beneath the chin to maintain one's coif while whizzing around in a convertible.

Then I was sent to Paris on assignment and there they were, everywhere, all tied in the most inventive ways, worn not for utility, but for style. I rushed home and started writing stories about them, while at the same time beginning my personal collection, which has reached embarrassing proportions today.

I could rhapsodize. Scarves are perhaps the simplest way to make a personal statement. Some sleight of hand takes practice, but, again, it's worth it.

Words of caution: scarves can be tied "old" or they can be tied "young." If you detect any hint of *dadame* (dowdy), quickly untie and start over.

It took me a while to get the hang of slinging a shawl around my shoulders and having it, by some metaphysical miracle, stay in place the way the ones Frenchwomen wear do. For beginners, an "important" brooch at the edge of the shoulder is not only a nice touch, but it also holds the construction in place. In time, like *moi-même*, you, too, will find just the right balance for the shawl.

Shawls do more than keep the upper body warm; they add the *je ne sais quoi* that transforms everything, from the classic jeans/blazer/white shirt combo to a little black dress, from simple to spectacular. A heavy, black cashmere number is very versatile; additional shawls are an ideal means to add color to a neutral wardrobe.

LINGERIE

Seriously, you didn't think anyone could write a book about Frenchwomen and not talk about lingerie, did you? No, I didn't think so.

Frenchwomen like to feel feminine. They like to feel confident. They like the feel of beautiful lingerie next to their skin. Furthermore, they adore the idea that they are wearing something beautiful and sensuous and very possibly unseen by anyone but themselves.

In my interviews and experimentation, I can confirm the hypothesis that underpinnings fulfill all those aspirations.

For years, the most exciting fripperies in my lingerie drawer were colorful—"color" being the operative word—sturdy, dependable, items that offered support (literally). I thought color was making a bold statement; obviously, it was not. I now have froufrou and daring pieces cohabiting alongside the mundane. My lacy/racy bits give me a covert frisson. I promise you, it's true. Also, some of them are every bit as supportive as their less embellished alternatives.

One fact is undeniable: lingerie is exciting, even if worn solely for our very private pleasure. Pretty unmentionables literally change a woman's attitude. They're powerful partially because they are our secret and they support the other part of our personalities that may, by necessity, hide beneath the clothes we wear.

As I sit in front of my computer, my lingerie—heather gray cotton, cute—matches, although it is neither sexy nor silky, but I am applying the basic rule every French mother teaches her daughter: never leave the house—or stay home for that matter—in lingerie that isn't color coordinated.

Remember how our mothers taught us to make sure our underwear was always clean? Our mothers were worried about accidents, whereas French mothers are perhaps more concerned with liaisons—a detail that speaks volumes about our cultural differences!

Chantal Thomass, one of France's most famous lingerie designers, realizes that some women don't care about what

Handle with Care

Madame Poupie Cadolle recommends that her underpinnings—haute couture and prêt-à-porter—be washed in warm water, by hand. "Shampoo is an excellent soap choice because it has no detergent ingredients," she said. "It's not the lace, which is sturdier than most of us think, but the elastic that is destroyed when women throw their lingerie into the machine."

she so dearly loves, but she believes that those who do care show that they understand lingerie's transforming effect. Thomass maintains that lingerie can make a woman sit, move, and even work differently.

She described her sultry collections as "feminine, seductive, comfortable, and impertinent" while emphasizing that comfort is essential. "Lingerie must make a woman feel good," she said.

One often hears and reads that Frenchwomen are addicted to silk lingerie, but when I asked my friends whether this was true, all but one said no.

Anne-Françoise said it's too much work: "hand wash, iron. I don't think so." She, like almost everyone I know, does own some, but the days of wearing it are in the past. As one friend pointed out, "Those were the days when we were young and had the time, or for some, we had someone who did the washing and ironing for us, and maybe we were wearing the ensembles more for someone else than for ourselves."

Geraldine, a longtime friend, said she has a small drawer with only silk bras, panties, and camisoles and that she wears them when she is feeling blue. Normally, she chooses her underwear from a larger drawer filled with easy-care, though pretty, pieces.

It's not difficult to find exquisite silk lingerie in Paris, but as far as I know, every emporium also offers more "reasonable" alternatives—that is, relatively reasonably priced and, most certainly, not requiring special care. Good silk lingerie is shockingly expensive and must be treated delicately.

Speaking of expensive, I had always heard about gorgeous custom-made lingerie being one of the great Parisian luxuries, but investigating the sources had never entered my mind—until I began my research for this book.

I picked up the phone and called the famous Madame Poupie Cadolle, purveyor and creator of astonishing lingerie. She is charm incarnate.

Her haute couture lingerie salon is hidden at the end of a long, dark corridor leading off the rue du Faubourg-Saint-Honoré. Madame Cadolle, dressed entirely in black, is *un peu ronde,* as the French say, with a pale complexion and straight shoulder-length hair the color of flax. She is a woman of a certain age, and she takes her mission of supporting our busts, reining in our waists, and lifting our derrieres very, very seriously. She also likes the idea that the wearing of her luxurious offerings can bring pleasure to the woman wearing them *and* the man in her life.

Sometimes, she confided, men come with their wives or girlfriends to choose ensembles. She was positively giddy over the idea that she could play a role in their romances.

Never mind. I was sitting in her peachy-blush bonbon of a boutique to find out why a woman would spend 650 euros (the least expensive bra) for bust support. At this question, Madame Cadolle became serious.

She abhors the pervasive trend in lingerie departments the world over that has women selecting their undergarments unarmed with crucial information that would help them have sublime bust lines and at the same time give them the support that will keep everything perky for the long term. She believes that most women are buying the wrong types of bras and doing an enormous disservice to their silhouettes. "It's a shame there are almost no trained personnel in most lingerie departments who can measure and assist women with their choices," she said.

That being the case, I asked her what we should look for when buying off-the-rack bras. This is what she told me:

- The cups should be rigid with seams that support the breasts.
- Contrary to what many women believe, straps must be solid and non-stretch to hold the bust in place.
- At the back, where the straps attach to the band, there should be some elastic.
- The band of the bra must sit low on the back. The higher the band on the back, the less support for the bust (think droop or sag). If the back rides up, the bust moves down.

Her haute couture salon is filled with every conceivable confection, including corsets of every imaginable color, nightgowns, camisoles, tap pants, high-tech—though gorgeous—nip-and-tuck constructions, robes, and garter belts.

Madame Cadolle lamented the fact that most women feel released from the constraints of garter belts. "They are so feminine, so sexy," she said. "Now they are mostly in the realm of fantasy (read: male fantasies)," she said. Brides like them, though, she added.

For the haute couture experience, as in pampered assistance without the three fittings and major investment, one can shop in Madame Cadolle's ready-to-wear boutique, a few steps away from the rarefied atmosphere of made-to-order. There, bra prices begin at about 150 euros.

VERNIS À ONGLES (NAIL POLISH)

Of course nail polish is an accessory. It's the best whimsical, budget-friendly detail ever invented. Why would cosmetic houses constantly introduce new colors, everything from gray and (almost) black to yellow, blue, and beyond, mingled with nuanced versions of the classics, if they didn't realize that some women cannot afford major investments in a new season, but chances are they can participate at the nail level?

Depending upon the condition of her hands, i.e., whether she has veins and spots, she can, if she dares, play with the spectrum of shades on the market. If she feels wild colors are too unkind on her, she always has her toes.

Among my friends, the majority stay on the pale pink side of the color wheel. When I venture into the town near our village, I see more daring, particularly among the women who own boutiques. They opt for grays, reds in every imaginable riff on the tone—from goth-deep Bordeaux to fresh, cheery cherries—and various takes on corals. They save the yellows and greens for their toes and usually match them with complementary sandals, leaving me with the impression that it's a fashion game as opposed to a personal statement. Last summer, one woman wore gray polish with silver sandals, a great look.

9

Enduring
Enchantments

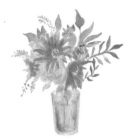

FORGET EXPIRATION DATES:
CHARM, GRACE, POISE, WIT, AND MORE

Frenchwomen, particularly those over forty, put as much effort into their comportment and their quality of life as they do into their personal styles. They actively and creatively construct their lifestyles with purpose and panache.

Over and over, they prove that what is pleasing to the eye is uplifting to the spirit, and that what is nourishing for the spirit is what makes life worth living.

Their attention to detail is reflected in everything they do. They bring the same refinement and rigor that they apply to themselves to their homes, their friendships, and—of paramount importance—the care and nurturing of their families.

Nothing is left to chance.

We know our subjects are captivating to the point of fascination on the outside. Now I would like to show you, and assure you, that they are equally, if not more, intriguing because of their character, their grace, and their charm.

THE ESSENCE OF BEAUTY

Style without substance is unacceptable, largely because it's boring, one-dimensional. In France, it's inadmissible to provoke *ennui*. Real style is built upon a solid foundation of informed intelligence, quick wit, and an impressive panoply of cultural references. One must hold her own in lively conversation. The essence of beauty is to continue educating oneself and constantly to learn something new. Simply put: these are the keys to eternal youth.

Nothing is more fascinating than a woman who piques the imagination with her clever, cultivated demeanor. Centuries before the modern concept of feminism arrived on French soil, Frenchwomen were masters of wresting power through influence, and much of their power grew out of their femininity, their poise, and, of course, their intelligence. History provides us with many examples of such women.

Long after her failing health made physical relations impossible, the Marquise de Pompadour remained a vital part of Louis XV's life. He turned to her for her gaiety, her "lightness," her counsel, and her trusted friendship. He found respite with her that he treasured throughout their nearly twenty-three years together. Well educated, pretty, and refined, the marquise painted, engraved, played the clavichord, and performed in plays that offered an escape for her king. She was reputed to have a lovely speaking and singing voice that enchanted him. The marquise also believed wholeheartedly in fun and diversion, and so she arranged lively dinner parties and card games to distract and amuse.

Her apartments were sumptuous, feminine, and filled with exquisite objects, flowers, delicate scents, and delicious delicacies. (She was the patron of the porcelain manufactory Sèvres, which created a magnificent rose porcelain in her honor. Her exquisite, albeit extravagant, taste is revered to this day.)

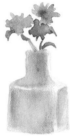

And she was, of course, magnificently turned out in the latest fashions, always choosing pastels that flattered her pale complexion. She was, after all, the main attraction upon the stage she had meticulously crafted for her king.

By gaining the king's confidence, she became his confidante and she exercised considerable influence on political decisions. Whether that was a good thing or a bad thing depends on which biographer one believes.

When she died of tuberculosis at forty-two, Louis XV, the great-grandson of Louis XIV, was devastated.

Another love story: it was the intelligence and kindness of Françoise d'Aubigné that attracted the Sun King, Louis XIV, to her.

After the death of his wife, María Teresa of Spain, Louis XIV married the fifty-one-year-old widow, to whom he gave the title Marquise de Maintenon, in a secret religious ceremony.

Historians say she was attractive, quite pious, gentle, and extremely bright. Before they married, the king passed hours in her company discussing politics, religion—there was much to discuss on that subject, since she herself was baptized a Catholic and partially raised a Protestant—and economics. At what point they became lovers has never been officially verified by historians, although many have pointed out that no matter how modest one's nature—and hers was reputed to be quite modest—when the king makes such a request, it's difficult to refuse.

It is said that she had enormous influence on her husband and was the force behind his fervent return to religion.

THE LEGACY OF THE SALON

Throughout the history of France, Frenchwomen were renowned and celebrated for their salons, where they entertained intellectuals, artists, writers, and bon vivants with the sole intention of provoking stimulating conversation, debate, amusing repartee, and lively exchanges of ideas. It was, in fact, a salon that brought Jeanne Poisson (who would come to be known as the Marquise de Pompadour) to the attention of the court. Her salon established her reputation in Paris as an intriguing woman of elegance and wit.

Intellectual stimulation is deeply embedded in French society. In fact, it has always been the highest form of seduction, and it continues to be so to this day. It would be unjust and prejudicial to insinuate that feminine wiles were these women's sole means of gaining entree into the world of power, but they were—and many claim they continue to be—part of a clever woman's repertoire of skills.

Many historians recognize French suffragettes at the time of the French Revolution as the first to float the notion of equality between the sexes.

Interestingly, however, Frenchwomen did not get the vote in France until 1944, and they actually cast their first ballots almost a year later to the day. For the sake of comparison, in the United States, the Nineteenth Amendment to the Constitution, which gave women the vote, was passed in 1920.

The seminal work of Simone de Beauvoir, *Le Deuxième Sexe* (*The Second Sex*), considered by many to be the ultimate treatise on modern feminism, was published in 1949. In it, she posed the question of the "Other," postulating that "existence precedes essence," and thus, "one is not born a woman, but becomes one." By extension, she maintained that existentialist philosophy should give her equal opportunity in society. She vigorously fought against preconceived ideas that men were superior to women and argued that women, despite centuries of submission to men, were perfectly capable of making intelligent, considered decisions.

THE POWER OF CONVERSATION

Often these fascinating elements of French history continue to be debated at dinner parties. They tend to be the things that make evenings unforgettable, and chances are that it will be a woman who introduces the subjects, just as in the days of their ancestors' salons.

I have actually attended dinner parties where arguments about which painter best captured the *real* Louis XIII or Louis XVI in his portrait dominated part of the meal. (I mean, really, have any of these people seen a recent photograph of the late kings?) My dinner companions verbally fenced over pot-au-feu and a breathtaking bottle of Chateau Latour Pauillac 2000 (the French do love to combine the simplicity of a peasant dish with the supreme sophistication of one of the best vintages of one of the world's best wines) about the size of noses and the folds of chins. How can one not love a French soirée?

Consider this: in a country where philosophy is a required subject in high school and has its own baccalaureate exam, how could one expect adults to forget the fun of the intellectual acrobatics involved in discussing and debating everything from the mundane to the esoteric?

Adults attacking philosophy exam questions is a great parlor game.

I can't help but wonder whether other countries have monthly philosophy magazines. France does, of course. The editorial purpose of *Philosophie* is to "make philosophy accessible to a large audience . . . through discussions of politics, society, science, economy, and the arts."

The only subject I've never heard discussed in social situations is religion. Religion is taboo because it could offend. One does not offend in polite French society. One may shock; indeed, that is expected, anticipated, and relished.

The French Are
DIFFERENT

For those of us whose mother tongue is English, the French language can present a minefield of misunderstandings, and not simply errors in grammar. (I'll never get my verbs in order.) Often words we would think of as synonyms are *faux amis*, or "false friends". "Education" is one of those words.

For us, education is what we learn in school. For the French, education is what one learns at home and in polite society: *politesse, savoir faire, courtoisie, moralité* and a vast appreciation of culture through exposure to art and history from regular visits to museums.

"Instruction" is what one absorbs in school. Culture, of course, is an important part of the educational system in France.

Recent subjects on high school philosophy tests asked students to argue their positions on such questions as:

- Would we be freer without the State?
- Are all beliefs contrary to reason?
- Is the sole reason for work to be useful?
- Is liberty menaced by equality?
- Is art less necessary than science?
- Does self-control depend upon self-knowledge?
- Does experiencing injustice teach one how to be just?

That leaves sex and politics on the table. Oh, yes, spicy Parisian gossip is always on the menu. Parisian gossip is as old as the kings' courts, and it's an essential ingredient in the heady cocktail that makes for scintillating exchanges.

Money, jobs, and social status, which many claim are never discussed freely the way they are in the United States, may be addressed, but these conversations adhere strictly to a far more circumspect social code. One mentions the weekend home in a chic corner of the countryside outside Paris, a family chateau, the chalet in Gstaad, the *petite maison* in Biarritz, titles, museum-worthy pieces of furniture "that have been in our family forever," *bijoux* passed down through the generations, etc.

Probably because I'm an American and we do not have the titled history of Europeans (although we do have our Mayflower royalty), I am surprised at not the disdain, exactly, but the sort of amazed and slightly pejorative appreciation of those who have made their success—read: riches—through their own employ and ambition. These *nouveau riche* success stories often make for lively gossip among those who have mainly managed to keep and occasionally grow their assets— or lost everything except for the crumbling chateau—as opposed to those who have earned it.

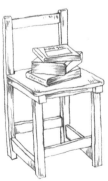

No matter what the subject ad-dressed in these conversations, one must be prepared and "educated." Frenchwomen are more than ready, and they love these encounters. What is more vibrant and seductive than a woman (or a man, for that matter) engaged in breathless debate? Age? What does age have to do with anything?

Conversation is sacred. It is an ageless, timeless pursuit shared and enjoyed with passion.

I do not know one Frenchwoman who does not rush out to see the latest exhibitions in Paris. Others seek out little-known museums and galleries and then share their discoveries with friends. They take their children and grandchildren to exhibitions, and then they discuss what they saw over lunch. In Paris, they see exposure to art, literature, theater, ballet, music, and food as being as necessary as breathing the air, and they believe that it is their duty to pass on their passions to the next generations. Often it is grandmothers who take on this joyful role. It gives them precious time with their grandchildren, and ultimately those moments are a priceless gift.

One friend of mine sits in on lectures at the Sorbonne. "I find them stimulating," she says. "Depending upon my mood, I choose a subject with which I am familiar and about which I want to learn more, or just the opposite, something I've never heard of before. When I discover something complicated and new, I regale my husband with my latest knowledge. He loves it. I think it's a little secret for a happy marriage—sharing an adventure."

I have friends who have season tickets to the opera and the ballet, while others prefer the theater, and just about everyone I know has the latest films on their to-see lists, including obscure offerings with subtitles—films that probably are only shown in the countries where they were produced and in small Paris art houses.

When was the last time you thought about seeing a film from Azerbaijan or Bangalore? My friend Edith and her husband seek out these low-budget productions whenever and wherever they can find them. Sometimes they're disappointed; often they're enthralled. I always get a report.

Slowly (and sadly), though, reality TV is usurping a portion of prime-time programming. Still, many prefer the brilliantly produced episodes of *Secrets d'Histoire*, a semi-regular series on one of the major channels (these types of programs are not relegated to obscure art and history channels in France) that presents the intrigue of the kings' courts, the love affairs, the affairs of state, the manipulations of the ambitious courtiers, the commissioning of some of the world's most exquisite works of art and decoration, the landscaping of Le Nôtre at Versailles and Vaux-le-Vicomte, the sensuous architecture of Louis Le Vau.

These programs unspool history like an irresistible fairy tale, with accounts from historians and relatives of the aristocrats in question recounting their families' stories, some reading aloud from historic letters and documents. The sagas are positively mesmerizing. And the bonus: we learn something. We're gathering anecdotes for our next dinner party conversation.

Actually, history and culture are everywhere. Not far from us, in the countryside west of Paris, relatives of

Lafayette have their weekend house. Since his descendants are friends of ours, I have been treated to a tour of their home, where portraits of Thomas Jefferson when he was ambassador to France mingle with priceless letters and documents framed and hung on the walls without concern for the potential damage wrought by sunlight, or the fluctuations in temperature that could put them in peril. My tour guides have been gracious and generous; the owners thought that as an American I would want to see some of our combined history. I was touched to the point of tears.

Since living in France and seeing the passion that history can evoke, I've always wondered why I was never once interested in the subject in school. Perhaps it's a question of how a story is told. And, heaven knows, the French know how to tell a good story.

THE IRRESISTIBLE POWER OF CHARM

Weaving a fascinating tale highlights yet another trait on which the French, both men and women, have built their stellar reputation: charm.

For many reasons, charm is the most enthralling characteristic in a Frenchwoman's repertoire. The word itself once led to an energetic Sunday luncheon conversation. I asked the men and the women present, "How do you define charm?" I don't know why I was surprised by the heated discussion that followed. The French language itself is a labyrinth of nuances and contradictions, and nowhere was that more evident than in the discourse that ensued.

I was told without equivocation by all present, "There is no comparison between a woman who has *du charme* and a *femme charmante*." Umm, okay, explain, please. Charm is charm, right?

Mais non. That would be too easy.

Forget about *du charme*. We're born with it—or not. It is the innate power to fascinate, to seduce. A child can have it; a woman of eighty-five will continue to have it. It is totally natural, and the woman who possesses *du charme* may not realize she has it until she reaches a certain age. One sees it in a gesture, in a look. It is a sort of mystical magic. One is drawn to *charme* like a moth to a flame. We're often powerless in its presence.

Catherine Nay, journalist and biographer (and gorgeous Frenchwoman), told me you can see *du charme* in an infant. She said, "I've seen it with my nephew. When he was a baby, before he could talk, he was completely bewitching. He was and is irresistible."

Perhaps it is what we would call charisma. It's rare and impossible to simulate. On the other hand, anyone can be *charmante* (charming), I'm told, and disarmingly so if they desire. It's an excellent substitute and completely attainable.

If it doesn't come naturally, my feeling is that, like everything else within these pages, it can be learned. Look directly into the eyes of the person to whom you are speaking. Offer compliments with extravagant generosity.

They must always be sincere. There is something kind and positive to be said about everyone. Listen intently, do not interrupt others in mid-conversation, and never forget that good manners are an extension of kindness.

I cannot emphasize enough the role of impeccable manners in French society—or maybe I have. In some instances manners take the shape of a formalized *gentillesse* (gentleness/kindness)—helping a timid guest participate in a conversation, for example. Under less intimate circumstances, there are rules of conduct that show respect without amity. These are elements of a Frenchwoman's charm that anyone can emulate.

As My-Reason-For-Living-In-France says, "There is something beautiful about every woman. Find it and tell her." He was born charming, but he has degrees of the characteristic depending upon his degree of friendship with or affinity for someone.

This is how the French define a charming woman of a certain age: she is vivacious, attentive, curious, cultured, lighthearted (seemingly), open, kind, amusing, and intelligent. Her manners are impeccable, and she knows how to, as the French say, *mettre les autres en valeur*, or make others feel important, interesting, valued. She asks questions and she *listens*.

Yes, there is coquetry in play, of course. Frenchwomen are born flirts,. They revel in seduction, usually of an innocent nature. It's a game, *très amusant*. Everyone knows the rules. I have passed some of the best moments of my life playing that game at French dinner parties.

I admit, for several years after I first arrived here and was in my early thirties, I was uncomfortable with these exchanges. I didn't realize they could be a simple social pastime to make an evening more piquant without the consequences that they seemed to imply. Once I caught on, though, I was hooked.

Am I saying that many of the mannerisms that were historically part of a woman's repertoire continue to exist today? Yes, I am. I think Frenchwomen in social situations tend to display the softer side of feminism, which in no way diminishes its effectiveness. The majority of my friends, ranging in age from their forties to their seventies, are feminists, but their battles with men are waged not at home, but rather in the public arena for equal pay, job opportunities, and positions in government and corporations.

This is an outsider's observation, confirmed by my friends. I could be wrong.

Frenchmen assured me that age has no importance for them. They added that their eyes, "like any healthy male's," are drawn fleetingly to a pretty young woman in a mini-skirt, but at a dinner party, if that pretty girl has nothing to say, they would prefer to be seated next to a woman who can entertain with her charm and wit.

The moment one is drawn into a woman's confidential web of sparkling conversation, no one is doing the math. Every man I interviewed, every man I know, including the one with whom I live, told me a façade is never enough to create enduring interest.

How can one not be captivated by a culture that celebrates the enduring enchantments of charm, wit, intelligence, and grace? And, furthermore, what could be more romantic than to realize that a beautiful mind is the perfect, ageless complement to a beautiful façade?

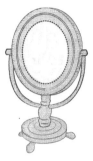

The Transformation

LA NOUVELLE MOI, A WORK IN PROGRESS

You may think that you are about to read the final installment in my transformative adventure, wherein I become more of *une femme d'un certain âge* than "a woman of a certain age." You understand the nuance, I trust—no matter which language we're using. I've got the age part under control, but there's no doubt about it, I'm convinced that what I've learned by living in France has greatly changed my life in many important ways.

This may be the epilogue, but my transformation is a continuing saga.

When I set out on my expedition, I was not trying to reinvent myself. Rather, I wanted to assimilate the best that I could wrest from the masters of looking vibrant and stylish at every age. An evolution, not a revolution, but, yes, with a French twist.

On so many levels, I know that I am not at all the same person I would have been had I never moved to France. The transformations that have occurred in my twenty-five-plus years in this country are as much attitudinal and philosophical as they are physical.

But let's start with the physical, shall we?

No doubt about it, I admit without equivocation that I love a fabulous façade. At the same time, I wanted to feel better, to have that certain *bien-être* or well-being that comes with taking good care of oneself on the inside. And, truthfully, I believe Frenchwomen tend to be more rigorous and successful on both fronts, and it shows on the outside.

That's why I set out on my journey. As you know, I've tried and rejected, avoided altogether, and outright usurped scores of their favorite rituals, routines, and realities.

I've succeeded, I've failed, and I've compromised, but believe me, I've done my best and the results have definitely justified the means. However, this is a war, not a battle—the defense tactics continue.

You can see the scenario coming into focus. I'm like a lab rat in pearls and perfume, and I can't get enough of this experiment because, as I suspected, the results are my new, improved theorem on elegance and élan.

A theorem is based on an idea accepted or proposed as true. *Et voilà!* I took, and continue to take, my preconceived notions and make them reality. Every day.

Don't think for an instant it's a piece of cake being French. It takes self-awareness and self-esteem to make an effort every day until effort becomes habit. Effortless elegance is an illusion. But here's the upside: these efforts are fun and fruitful. The rewards are obvious. When I look in the mirror, I see great skin; perfectly cut, swingy hair; a slimmer figure—no one expects an *haricot vert* (string bean) body, least of all me; regal posture; and a renewed self-possession that radiates confidence. You'll see that it's a win-win. When we take the absolute best care of ourselves, the bonus is looking and feeling younger, healthier, chic, and *bien dans notre peau*.

Throughout my endeavor, discipline and dedication have been paramount on my mind, and I've discovered living by these codes has given me a new freedom.

I'm willing to exfoliate with care and vigor while in the shower and slather on some lotion thereafter, but the anti-cellulite, drainage products require true dedication.

When I was lucky enough to be treated to ninety-minute drainage/anti-cellulite massages at the Clarins Institute, it was heaven, but these are not one-off treatments. To see appreciable results, it's necessary to have regular massages, which I assure you would not be a burden on the body—but the budget is another story.

ON THE RECORD: I have not given up, because I made a promise, but it's not easy. I think this is a ritual that will take more than a month or two to become a habit.

Similarly, for *un ventre plat*, a flat stomach, I'm not even pretending to rub any gels, creams, or lotions on that part of my body. Thank goodness my pharmacist is a friend and told me to save my money and invest in yoga classes. I did; she was right.

Self-tanners were an absolute catastrophe for me, and this was not from lack of desire or good intentions. For years I simply couldn't get it right—streaks and brown toenails. Frenchwomen never get it wrong. The mere idea was always thrilling; tanned legs year-round are sublimely seductive. The fact that legs look thinner and younger when *bronzées*—self-tanner is a great cover-up for unsightly spots and veins—made the notion even more appealing. After practicing, not every day you understand, but often, for a very long time, I finally mastered the technique. Self-tanning is one of my greatest triumphs.

Predictably, there are the gray areas in my quest, the compromises, the *laisser-aller*. As I sit here in front of my computer, I have on zero makeup, unthinkable for a Frenchwoman. Even though I have no plans to leave the house today, I can't be 100 percent certain that the water-meter man won't come to the door or our charming postal lady won't deliver a package. Yikes! What would they think? Who would they tell? Why do I care?

However, on rising this morning, I sprayed my face with an *eau thermale* for delicate skin (*peaux sensibles*) and applied my amazing anti-age day serum, followed by a cream that boasts the same promise, and thus I presume they're doing their jobs as I work. My hair is held back with a headband, the ultimate French cradle-to-grave, bad-hair-day accessory. I actually haven't had a bad hair day in years. I always wear a headband or put my hair in a ponytail when I work. For some psychological reason, I need my hair to be up, up, and away when I write.

My eyelashes are curled, and on my lips I have a lightly tinted lip balm that has the slightest hint of color and, best of all, a magically subtle, sparkly effect. Maybe this means that, technically, I'm not without a hint of artifice.

I'm wearing a light gray Uniqlo T-shirt, my cute cashmere Bompard pullover—black with light and dark gray trim at neck and sleeves—and I am not wearing sweats or my pajama bottoms, but rather a pair of pinstripe gray flannel H&M trousers with a smidge of stretch fabric. Comfortable or not, I have yet to start wearing pants with elastic waists. Frenchwomen of a certain age—and as we all know, I like to follow their lead when and where I can—use their skirt and trouser buttons to tell them when to pull back on the calories.

So do I.

MY ACCESSORIES: a multi-gray herringbone wool-and-cashmere scarf, looped tightly around my neck—*à la française*—and gold *créole* earrings; my feet are snug in a pair of my husband's black, gray, and red argyle socks—you can see I've got a theme going here—and shod in black suede loafers. (If I were to leave the house I would apply blush, recurl my eyelashes with the world's greatest implement from Shu Uemura, and whisk on some mascara.)

My toenails are painted a gorgeous Fuchsia Provoc. My fingernails are polished with Delicacy by Essie, a low-maintenance barely there hint of color.

I've also spritzed a soupçon of one of my favorite fragrances, Parfum d'Hermès, on my nape and my wrists, as I do every day no matter what. The nape is for when My-

Reason-For-Living-In-France gives me a kiss there, and the wrists are for me.

My underwear, though not alluring, matches. Today the duo is a deep red, but it does not feature any lace or fancy trim. Color is making my secret statement.

THE QUESTION BEGS TO BE POSED: before moving to France, would I have made these miniscule efforts to work alone in my home office without a visit from anyone other than my dogs? Probably not, but here's the difference: it is no longer the slightest effort to "pull myself together," and over time I have realized dressing up is a joy.

I have to admit, I've always loved to take as much time as possible bathing, making up, planning and laying out my clothes and accessories, and getting dressed for occasions. For me, anticipation and preparation are part of the fun. Even "dressed down," I am no longer comfortable throwing on any old mismatched whatever that may or may not be wrinkled, along with underwear that deserves to be tossed. It has no appeal. It doesn't *feel* right. I don't need an occasion to get dressed. Getting up and getting out there is all the reason I require.

Now, what about the psychological, the philosophical? As much as I appreciate Frenchwomen for their beauty esthetic, I perhaps admire them equally for their philosophy of life. They are grounded in reality, which does not preclude passion or romance, but does guarantee a certain healthy respite from despair and a profound appreciation for life in general.

I see a constant, conscientious effort to emphasize the positive in relationships.

Since France is a country that reveres its philosophers, and where philosophy is a required subject in high school, it seems only logical that one tends to see a more global, abstract view of human behavior here. It's a notion I find exceedingly appealing in theory and, when not in the heat of an unpleasant moment, I try to look at the bigger picture and to be more forgiving. It's not always easy, but without being too Pollyanna-ish about the approach, I've found it leaves me feeling more generous and less churlish. It takes more energy to be unkind and spiteful than it does to be kind.

Moving right along . . . I shall now share with you a list—you know how I love lists—of the tangible and intangible things I do regularly that I believe are a direct result of living in France:

- More isn't necessarily more. More is often disappointing, sometimes even depressing.
- Accentuate the positive in mind and body.
- Every woman must have her trusted, talented army of enablers (her seamstress, hairstylist, shoe person, dermatologist, etc.)
- Keep a few secrets.
- Since we're our own best investments, it's essential to find "me" time.
- Learning to say no is liberating. Sometimes it takes practice, but overextending ourselves can make us miserable and bitter.
- The auxiliary rule of the above: We are not in a popularity contest. We cannot please all of the

people all of the time. Not everyone will like us, *c'est la vie*.

- Wear perfume every day, just because.
- Personal favorite: polish your toenails throughout the year. I get a special frisson of delight from this oh-so-simple habit.
- Budget for items and services that give the best return on investment: haircuts and hair color, two or three great bags, good shoes.
- Forget about advertising promises. Often the pharmacy has the best beauty products at reasonable prices.
- A dermatologist is a necessity, not a luxury.
- Organization conquers stress and chaos.
- Effort in equals pleasure out. And that includes everything from a beautifully set dinner table, every day, and healthful meals to bouquets scattered about the house and a fire in the fireplace.
- Pause and think before reacting to anything, be it an impulse purchase, a second *macaron*, or an unkind retort.
- Conversation need not be a lost art.
- Wear the same clothes you feel and look good in over and over. They give you confidence and power. Quality over quantity.
- Rethink lingerie.
- Cheap shoes are expensive.
- If we're on a diet, we don't need to tell everyone we meet. The results speak louder than words.

- Better than the theory of relativity is the double-E maxim: Excess + Exception = zero weight gain, no guilt, and a heightened sense of pleasure. As in, Frenchwomen look at the occasional piece of chocolate cake as fit for a *fête*, meaning they anticipate it and enjoy it, but don't make it a habit.
- A woman can *never* own too many scarves.
- Discipline will set you free.

WHAT, THEN, IS THE ULTIMATE BEAUTY SECRET?

When I asked every Frenchwoman I know what they think the secret to youthful beauty is, no matter what their age, almost every one said, "*l'amour*." They must be onto something because a recent magazine article talked about the mind/body/skin benefits of making love.

More than that, though (or, as well as that, if we're lucky), they added the following to the formula: good food; some wine; exercise; constant mental stimulation; relaxation; deep friendships; and a general philosophy of life that puts stress, worries, and aging into perspective.

Ç'est la vie, that's life, is more than a casually meaningless expression in France. Often when I hear someone declare, *ç'est la vie,* it is in acceptance of a difficult moment, because life, by definition, has its joys and sorrows, but it never precludes a determined effort on the part of Frenchwomen, particularly those of a certain age, to create joy and beauty wherever and whenever they can.

What could be more youth and beauty enhancing than deciding to make one's life as positive and purposeful as possible?

In the end, it's not about anti-aging. No matter what we do, time marches on. It's all about taking care of ourselves, improving our minds as well as our spirits (and our style, of course). Style is the ageless extension of one's personality. Like Frenchwomen, I never think I'm not worth the effort, that nobody cares or notices me. I care, and others do as well. After all, looking the best we can is every woman's ultimate natural depression remedy. I wish you the best of luck on your journey!

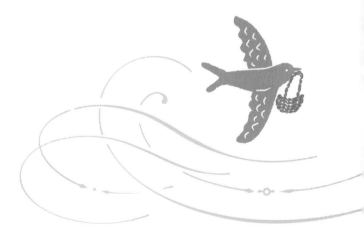

ACKNOWLEDGMENTS

Where to begin?

Writing this book was one of the most extraordinary experiences of my life. I had such fun in my interviews and so appreciate the time everyone took to explain, and in some cases to pamper me—think massages, makeup lessons, wardrobe ideas—as I did my research.

First, let me thank you for reading my book. I hope you enjoy reading it as much as I enjoyed writing it.

Now, let me tell you about the people who made it all possible . . .

Without my dear, dear friend Betty Lou Phillips, this book would not have existed. It's a long story, but suffice it to say that I am eternally grateful for her help and encouragement.

Betty Lou called a friend of hers, who introduced me to Lauren Galit, who is now my agent. Lauren is the type of agent another friend (and author) told me no longer exists, a "hands-on"—which at times included "hand-holding" —professional. Through the proposal process she gave me pep talks and reality checks. She knows how much I value her honesty and friendship.

From day one, Rizzoli was the publisher of my dreams, which sometimes really do come true. Thrilled would be an understatement when Kathleen Jayes, my editor, told me Rizzoli wanted to publish my book. Working with Kathleen was a pleasure and her intelligent, crisp, delicate editing made this book so much better. I am so very, very grateful to her.

Then there are the friends who "filled in" by writing posts for my blog, and who read sketchy attempts at the proposal, rough chapters of the book, and on and on. Foremost, is my darling Marsi Buckmelter, who was there from the very beginning of not only the book process, but also the blog. Thank you also to the absolutely delightful Janice Rigs for all of her invaluable help and kind words. Debra Wolf, you have been so very supportive and are a true friend. Deb Chase, your expertise was invaluable.

Merci!

A special thank you to Sujean Rim for her adorable cover illustration and to LeAnna Weller Smith for her creative art direction.

Ah, and my blogging friends, *merci mille fois* for writing blog posts and sending e-mails full of encouragement, support, and kindness. You are wonderful. I can never tell you enough how much you mean to me.

More friends who are important to me for all the reasons they know: Robert Olen Butler, Art Joinnides, Trisha Macolm, Philip Miller, Alice Bumgartner, James Washburn, and Sarah Burningham.

And, a very special thank you to one of my best friends in the world, Judy Diebolt, for always being there, for always understanding, for everything.

Thank you as well to Will Fletcher, my charming, hilarious son-in-law and extremely talented writer.

And always, always to the great loves of my life: Alexandre and Andrea, nothing would be possible without you.

"We are always
the same
age inside."

—GERTRUDE STEIN